Emotional Vampires and Your Hormones

An Holisitic Physician's View on How Stress Affects Your Well-Being and What You Can Do About It

ALAN J. SAULT MD, ABHM

BALBOA.
PRESS
A DIVISION OF HAY HOUSE

Balboa Press books may be ordered through booksellers or by contacting:

Balboa Press
A Division of Hay House
1663 Liberty Drive
Bloomington, IN 47403
www.balboapress.com
1-(877) 407-4847

Because of the dynamic nature of the Internet, any web addresses or links contained in this book may have changed since publication and may no longer be valid. The views expressed in this work are solely those of the author and do not necessarily reflect the views of the publisher, and the publisher hereby disclaims any responsibility for them.

The author of this book does not dispense medical advice or prescribe the use of any technique as a form of treatment for physical, emotional, or medical problems without the advice of a physician, either directly or indirectly. The intent of the author is only to offer information of a general nature to help you in your quest for emotional and spiritual well-being. In the event you use any of the information in this book for yourself, which is your constitutional right, the author and the publisher assume no responsibility for your actions.

Any people depicted in stock imagery provided by Thinkstock are models, and such images are being used for illustrative purposes only.
Certain stock imagery © Thinkstock.

Printed in the United States of America.

ISBN: 978-1-4525-8175-0 (sc)
ISBN: 978-1-4525-8176-7 (e)

Library of Congress Control Number: 2013916350

Balboa Press rev. date: 11/26/2013

I dedicate this book to my wife, Jennifer; who has dedicated so much of her patience and knowledge to me. Without her spirituality and teaching me the connection of mind-body-spirit I would not be on this path to teach others of these connections and how stress relates to dis-ease.

TABLE OF CONTENTS

PREFACE

My Autobiography of How and Why I Became an Expert
and Compassionate Holistic Physician

AFTER GRADUATING MEDICAL SCHOOL AND finishing my internship,
I decided to specialize in Emergency Medicine at Bowman Gray
School of Medicine at Wake Forest University in North Carolina.
I was chief resident for two years before I began working in a
200-patient per day emergency department. I certainly saw all there
is on the black side of human behavior, but also some really neat
people both as patients and comrades. I also worked as a medical
examiner, which was not always as romantic a position as is depicted
on TV. I did all of this for 15 years before transitioning to General
Medicine while teaching at the medical school. It was during this
time of seeing between 30-100 clients per day that I started realizing
how much I was missing by seeing a huge number of patients and
quickly diagnosing and treating them with pharmaceuticals. I
realized that seeing the same clients, for the same or related diseases, happened because I did not have the time to identify the cause
of their ailments, but was instead only treating signs and symptoms. I
also had numerous sports injuries of my own that were not improving
as my colleagues were treating my signs and symptoms rather than
identifying the root cause of the problems.

I was active in many sports, and back then I was doing full
contact karate and had fifteen years of karate experience under my
belt. After a fight my wife would do Reiki on me and in 15 minutes

I would feel great. Of course when I went in to teach the emergency residents with my black eye, they just figured that was weird Sault and he was probably on codeine, and it was the Reiki that was the cure and not the opioids. My wife, Jennifer is a pacifist and one night she said she would not perform Reiki on me anymore. At the time, I did not know anything about universal energies, only that Reiki worked. Therefore, I took a Reiki course so I could administer Reiki to myself. It was from this Reiki that I started to learn about universal energies that we all possess.

Because my injuries were not improving with the treatment plans recommended by colleagues, I started investigating alternative healing methods and, with time and employing these methods, I began doing better. Pretty soon I was working part time in a small office treating patients with alternative medicine. I started listening to my very spiritually evolved wife and became more interested in mind-body-spirit medicine, which, to me, is different than alternative medicine. Alternative medicine is using supplements and/or other types of healing methods other than western medical treatments. Holistic medicine involves thinking and combining mind-body-spirit, alternative treatments, and when necessary western medicine. Included in holistic medicine is the search for the underlying cause of sickness, which is the curative part of medicine. Fortunately I have the knowledge to use or combine traditional western medicine when I deem it necessary, which is not too often. Following this path and seeing the relationship to dis-ease, stress and hormones I began working with bio-identical hormones and have been practicing anti-aging medicine for about 15 years.

When I was 65 I had a terrible headache for a week. It was like a hot poker going through the right side of my forehead. I went to work anyway because I had so many chronically ill patients who were depending on me. After 5 days of severe pain I had an MRI that showed two bleeding spots in the right side of my head. I went to the ED and, after another MRI (which I asked to defer because I had one earlier in the day); they diagnosed me with a bleed in the frontal right lobe of my brain. The ED physician did not know why I had the bleed so I was started on prednisone to reduce swelling at the site and to see if it was cancer. When I entered the ED my blood pressure was 180/120 and when they went to set up the MRI my wife did hypnosis on me. When they returned my blood pressure was120/70—without medicine! This is the good part of the story. Ironically, in the morning at the ED, there was a doctor standing over my bed that was one of the doctors I trained 20 years ago.

I was sent home on prednisone to see when the swelling came down so they could rule out a tumor versus a hemorrhage, but no reason for the bleed was diagnosed. Within three days I was back in the ED because I could not breathe. When they did a scan of my lungs they found what is called a saddle embolus, which are clots in both pulmonary arteries. About 94% of people with a saddle embolus in the pulmonary arteries die with this suddenly. I also had blood clots in my spleen and a hole in my upper heart chambers. The doctors, about 4 at this time, were not sure what to do; if they gave me anticoagulants to keep my blood from clotting I might bleed into my brain, but if they did not I might throw another clot and die. They put me on a morphine drip and heparin. The pain was excruciating for days, even with the morphine. Jennifer stayed with me night and day and meditated, as did other friends. Eventually I seemed better and they let me go home on Coumadin. I feared being on Coumadin, as much as I feared more blood clots due to the medication's side effects. Days later I returned to the ED with the same problem—I could not breathe—and I was admitted to the hospital again. Same problem, same death prognosis, same treatment. This time I had six doctors and even more blood tests done. Special blood tests were sent to the Mayo Clinic and these results showed a pretty new clotting disorder that is genetic but does not show up until a person is in the 50s-60s range. The story goes on and on. I had to give up my practice and we had huge medical bills and with insurance that did not cover a lot of it. Jennifer used up all the savings on doctors' and hospital bills and me not working.

My sister has the same gene (Gr2001A), which is what the Mayo Clinic tests identified in me, but she does not get stressed about little things—I do! I am positive that it was stress that brought out this predisposition because for years I worked long hours and a high percentage of this was for people that could not pay. I tell you my personal story to explain why I wrote *Emotional Vampires and Your Hormones: An Holistic Physician's View on How Stress Affects Your Well-Being and What You Can Do About It.*

Jennifer and I give seminars on stress and its relationship to illness and well-being. Our seminars are unique because I, as an MD, teach the medical part—the physiology of how stress affects, for example, the thyroid, and are responsible for diabetes and cardiovascular disease, etc. Jennifer, as a psychoanalyst with degrees in hypnotherapy and interactive guided imagery, teaches the alleviation of stress by taking the audience through techniques they can use at home.

ACKNOWLEDGEMENTS

I BELIEVE THIS BOOK WILL help many people, but this book only came about because I needed lots of help in the writing. The first one to thank is my teacher. She was the person to teach me about spirituality, stress and its role in dis-ease, a lot of the healing powers of alternative medicine, the Universe and still trying to teach me about unconditional-nonjudgmental love. Yes I am talking about my wife Jennifer Sault MFA, MS/Eds, LMHC. Not an easy task since I was so entrenched in allopathic medicine and teaching and practicing it at the Bowman Gray School of Medicine.

Next is another powerful woman—my editor—Jennifer Garrett Smith. She took on a jigsaw puzzle of a book and never complained. Her husband Mark Smith supporting her and me with his insights, his mother and my friend Myra Grozinger (who did the illustrations with me) and the Smiths' son Ivan who designed and redesigned the cover many times until we were satisfied. A real family of friends.

Of course, there is the physician that I give credit to saving my life, the hematologist-oncologist Steven Mamus M.D. Although I had six physicians working on my clotting disorder he was the one that figured out the cause, treated me and has become a caring friend.

I would like to thank all of the authors whose books and articles have taught me so much and stimulated me but that would be a novel in itself. But there are few that I would like to mention because, besides giving me insights to new paths and knowledge, maybe some of the readers will read their books in the entirety: Peter Kash et el *Freedom from Disease*; Bruce Lipton, Ph.D. *The Biology of Belief*; and

William Ferril M.D; the first person to help me integrate how all the hormones work like a symphony in his book *The Body Heals*. Another wonderful teacher and author is James L. Wilson author of *Adrenal Fatigue: The 21st Century Stress Syndrome.*

There was a time in my life that I was really exasperated with conventional—allopathic medicine. The organizations that inspired, reenergized my love of medicine, and taught me so much in complimentary medicine are the American College for the Advancement of Medicine (ACAM) and the American College of Holistic Medicine (ACHM). The latter along with my wife, Jennifer, taught me the relationship in medicine of mind, body, and spirit. I was in the very first group of physicians to take and pass their board certification for holistic medicine. Thanks to both groups for saving me and hundreds of my patients.

My granddaughter Izabella has taught me so much about laughing as a child, which is a great stress reliever. I thank her wonderful parents Nancy and my son Wayne Sault for not only bringing her into this world but also for being continuously present in my life with happiness and reminding me of giving unconditional love.

CHAPTER 1

What is an Emotional Vampire?

EMOTIONAL VAMPIRES ARE HUGE BAT-LIKE creatures that can turn into smoke. They sneak under your bedroom door at night and suck your blood. No? Well, not really, but emotional vampires are just as insidious. I define emotional vampires as the people, events, memories, environmental toxins, pace of life, and other elements of our current way of living that create increased, abnormal levels of stress that suck the life energy out of us. The terms normal and abnormal have nothing to do with what has become common or prevalent, but everything to do with the way our bodies are designed to function.

Imagine that you can travel back in time to the dawn of humankind; that you are hairy with short, strong limbs and dirty bare feet. You are dressed in animal skins that likely smell more than a bit raunchy. Your home is a cave, shared with others in your family and community. There are children running about and adults cooking, scraping skins, or making tools. At the entrance to the cave is a fire for warmth and protection and at the back of the cave are paintings depicting your spiritual beliefs or activities of daily life. You are homosapiens, the latest evolutionary model of Man. Homo sapiens means wise or thinking man because of the size of the cerebral cortex, which is the thinking part of the brain.

Now imagine that you are out hunting, carrying tools and weapons that you have made yourself—a stone ax or a stout stick that you have

1

sharpened to a point and hardened in the fire. Most of the animals you hunt are stronger, bigger, and faster than you are, so you hunt cooperatively with the other members of the group. Suddenly, you hear a low growl behind you and very carefully you turn your head to look over your shoulder. There is a huge saber-toothed tiger poised to attack. Its teeth are bared; its fangs are about six inches long and dripping saliva. Its eyes glow yellow and mean and they're looking straight at you.

You have two choices: you can fight it or you can run away. Immediately, without conscious thought, your body prepares you to do one or the other. A variety of hormones are released into the bloodstream that sends signals to just about every system in your body in preparation for physical action. As you watch the tiger you are aware, perhaps, that your breathing has quickened and your heart is pounding, though you don't stop to figure out why.

Your breathing quickens to take in more oxygen as your heart rate and blood pressure increase to pump the oxygen around the body for extra energy. There are a lot of other things going on in your body that you are not aware of.

You are shutting down non-essential functions such as digestion, which is not a priority when your life is at stake.

Your body is taking blood away from non-essential areas—such as the skin—and pumping that extra blood into the large muscles of your arms and legs.

Your liver is dumping its stored glucose into the bloodstream to give you extra energy.

Perhaps you and your group decide to fight the tiger or you decide to run. Either way, if you're successful, the burst of physical activity is a signal to your body to bring everything back to normal. Your heart rate slows down, digestion picks up where it left off, blood sugar levels stabilize, and blood pressure comes back to normal. If you're not successful you do not have to worry about stress any more. Or anything else, ever again.

It is now a hundred thousand years later. There are not any saber-toothed tigers around, but your body has not changed and it responds to stress in the same way, though the stressors we have to deal with today are very different. The stress response still prepares the body for physical action, even if the stressor is an unreasonable boss, a dysfunctional relationship, time pressure, financial problems, fear of terrorists.

None of these requires that we fight something or run away from it, but when the body perceives a stressor its response is still to prepare for a physical reaction as if there were no difference between a saber-toothed tiger and a work deadline. If we don't do something to relieve the stress the body never gets the signal to return to normal; it stays on high alert. What we as a society are experiencing today are chronic levels of stress that, over time, create or contribute to illness. Among the effects of the stress response are:

Digestion shuts down, so chronic levels of stress create problems in the digestive system: trouble swallowing, acid reflux, indigestion, diarrhea or constipation.

Heart rate and blood pressure increase, so chronic levels of stress create problems in the circulatory system: hypertension, strokes, and heart disease.

Stored glucose is dumped into the blood stream, so chronic levels of stress contribute to disorders related to sugar imbalance: diabetes and hypoglycemia.

The heightened awareness of the stress response can cause anxiety, headaches, muscle tension and insomnia.

Anxiety and stress can cause sexual dysfunction.

Chronic stress weakens the immune system, the body's defense system, so stress is a factor in physical illness because it lowers our resistance. If it gets bad enough or lasts long enough the body breaks down.

Stress creates imbalances in the hormonal systems of the body, which is the principal focus of this book.

We often don't even realize how stressed we are. Often, when I would ask patients about the stress in their lives they would say, "Oh no, there's nothing special going on." When I probed a little deeper I might find that they were the sole caretaker for a bedridden parent, and a teenage child just got a DUI, or the spouse was just laid off, and so on. That's the way our lives are, and we are so used to it that we think it's normal. But it's not normal for our bodies.

A common response to what feels like the uncontrollable stress in our lives is anger, a generalized anger at the whole world sometimes. We feel helpless to change or control the hamster wheel that we're running on. Anger has been identified as the number one risk factor in heart disease, a bigger risk than LDL cholesterol levels, smoking, obesity, lack of exercise; of all the risk factors we hear so much about, anger tops the list.

Researchers at the American Institute of Stress estimate that between 75 and 90 percent of all visits to health-care providers result from stress-related disorders. Stress is costing us in quality of life, in illness and disease, in money for health care, and in lost productivity.

RESPONSE TO STRESS IS INDIVIDUAL

Response to stress is an individual one; something that really freaks out one person may be no big deal for another. It is not the stress itself that's the problem but how we cope with it. If something is a source of stress for you, it doesn't matter how many times or how many people tell you it's no big deal.

We tend to think of stress as a negative, but stress can be a great motivator that nudges us to be more productive. Do you, or someone you know, find that creativity and productivity flow more easily when you have a deadline? It is often the difference in perception that causes some stress to be good stress (eustress) rather than bad stress (distress). Think about the lives of symphony conductors, for example. They work long hours, travel constantly, deal with prima donnas and sensitive artists, yet often live long and productive lives. Arturo Toscanini conducted his last concert when he was 87; Arthur Fiedler of the Boston Pops lived to be 105; Leopold Stokowski conducted the London Symphony Orchestra for over 60 years, and signed a contract with Columbia Records when he was 94.

If some of us lived like that—long hours, constant travel, temperamental people throwing tantrums all over the place—we would be basket cases. But for them their stressful lives were positive motivators; what for us might feel like overwhelming pressures, for them were perceived as stimulating, exciting, and fulfilling. They enjoyed what they were doing; they had pride of accomplishment, the approval of their peers, the applause of the audience, all positive stresses that contributed to productivity and life satisfaction.

Changing the way we think about various stresses in our lives can make a huge difference in our ability to respond to them in positive ways.

TIMING

Timing also has an impact on the way stress affects us. We are all more vulnerable at some times than others, especially if we are already dealing with something else. Something that's no big deal this week may tip you over the edge next week, just because of where you are and how you are feeling at that particular time. It's not a good idea to think about moving to a new town and starting a new job just after going through a divorce, for example.

ANY CHANGE IS STRESSFUL

Stress is a fact of life. The big things are obvious: death of a loved one, divorce, illness, getting fired, foreclosure and so on. But in fact change of any kind is a source of stress, positive or negative. Getting divorced is stressful, but so is getting married. Losing your job is stressful, but so is getting a promotion.

Holmes and Rahe are two research psychologists who developed a scale for rating stressful events. At the top of the list is the death of a spouse and second is divorce. Ninth is marital reconciliation while sixteenth is a change in financial state. Notice it says change, so either losing money or gaining money is perceived by the body as equally stressful.

Avoiding stress is impossible. Even if you had unlimited money and resources you would still have to deal with people, computers, government regulations, family members, environmental toxins, and so on. Stress is a fact of life, which begins in early childhood and never lets up. We have learned to accept it, and are often unaware that the levels of stress in modern life are injurious to our mental and physical health.

Karen came into my office complaining of volatile mood swings, fatigue, lethargy, depressed libido, and forgetfulness. She was surprised when I asked her about the stress in her life instead of writing her a prescription, but once she started to talk it was as if she had been waiting all her life for an opportunity to let out all the dammed up energy of her frustrations.

She learned very early in life, both from her mother's example and from the many overt and covert messages from other family members and her culture, that it was her job to be a caretaker and a peacemaker. By the time I saw her she was in her forties, had a full time job as a restaurant manager and was caring for a home, two teenage children, and a workaholic husband. She also spent several hours a week helping her elderly parents.

It was a revelation to Karen that the stress in her life was contributing directly to her physical symptoms.

Steve was a 45 year old white male suffering from shortness of breath, depressed sexual drive, fatigue and headaches, especially in his neck and the back of his head. He said he was getting angry over little things that would not have bothered him before. He, too, expected a prescription for his symptoms, but unlike Karen was not at first willing to spend any time talking about the general conditions of his life. He had been taught at a very early age that "complaining" was a sign of weakness. He was not at all interested in learning how to change his lifestyle. Not until his first heart attack, anyway.

One of the stressors that we grow up with are the double messages we get both from caretakers and society at large about what our role is supposed to be. A little girl may be called a princess from the moment she emerges from the womb and given overt and covert messages that she deserves to be taken care of. She may be acculturated to believe it is not feminine to express, or even feel, anger. She may not know how to express or take care of her own needs if she has been taught to put others first, and that it is feminine and attractive to be dependent on the decision-making of others. A male child as a toddler may be cuddled when he falls, but then at around age four or five if he falls and cries he is told that big boys do not cry. He may be told that he should be kind to others but also that he should watch his back and not be too trusting, a double message which later in life can cause relationship stresses.

The point is that stress starts very early but unobtrusively, and it is compounded by a relatively new stressor of which we are only just beginning to appreciate the dimensions: environmental toxins.

Phthalates (estrogen mimickers) have crept into widespread use over the past several decades. Their intentional uses include softeners of plastics, oily substances in perfumes, additives to hairsprays, lubricants and wood finishers. Their use has become so widespread—about a billion pounds per year are produced worldwide—that they can contaminate just about anything.

We are exposed to phthalates from plastics almost from birth from plastic formula bottles, plastic bed sheets, nipples and bottles, which leech into the soluble liquid in the bottle, diapers, toys and so forth. Plastics containing phthalates are estrogen mimics that take up the receptor sites of cells that should be for natural estrogen; they give off, or outgas, chemicals that interfere with or stimulate the estrogen receptors and therefore negatively influence estrogen balance.

We can see the effects of this in the early maturation of girls, who may now begin their menses as early as age nine, though plastic is not the only culprit in this situation. Many of the animals that produce our milk and meat are fed hormones to stimulate growth and production, and these hormones that are passed on when we ingest the meat and milk products. Just this morning a medical news note was on my computer by pediatricians noting that there seems to be not only in girls under 8 but also boys an increase in pre-puberty maturation with hair growth. They go through some questionable causes by never mention hormonal dairy and meats and phthalates (estrogen mimickers). They infer that this could become the normal. Being normal does not make it healthy. Plastic estrogen mimics can be measured in supermarket foods that are packaged in plastic. As adults we continue to be contaminated by phthalates in food and other environmental sources such as those mentioned previously. There is a little triangle at the bottom of each plastic bottle that denotes how safe the plastic is. If the triangle is a #2, 4 or 6 it is relatively safe with #6 being the best.

Lead used to be a major environmental stressor, contributing to many physical and mental problems in children. We worked long and hard to safeguard our children from lead exposure and passed laws and regulations to protect them only to discover that toys and other products manufactured abroad do not have to follow our rules.

Time Magazine reported that mercury, mostly from coal burning, is making many birds infertile and is killing whole species. We, of course, breathe the same air and drink the same water. We know that an expectant mother can pass mercury to her fetus and that mercury has toxic effects on the brain and other organs yet we continue to use mercury (thimerosal) as a preservative in childhood vaccines and the flu vaccines.

Other toxic heavy metals in the environment are:

Cadmium from cadmium-nickel batteries, cigarettes, waste sites, and smelting of metals. Cadmium can affect the kidneys and increases the risk of lung cancer, liver problems, and bone fractures. It is linked to prostate cancer and cardiovascular illness.

Aluminum, potentially one of the contributors to Alzheimer's disease, is used in cosmetics and cooking utensils.

Arsenic has been a well-known poison for centuries yet is found in the treated lumber used to build children's playgrounds. In some places the arsenic-treated playground structures have been dismantled and ground into mulch that the children walk on. Big improvement. Arsenic is also found in some soil where food is grown—most recently in rice.

We know that each of these heavy metals is toxic in certain concentrations, but as yet there is little research on the synergistic effect of ingesting all of them, even when the levels of each one are of a non-threatening concentration. Genetically some people can handle a heavy metal load of one type better than others, but the cumulative load may be too much.

In addition, we breathe in petrochemicals and toluene from carpets, we ingest herbicides, pesticides and insecticides; our water systems tax our bodies with fluoride—which can hurt the teeth (dental fluorosis), bones, and thyroid gland—and chloride, which can displace the iodide needed by the thyroid. You can search the Internet for scientific articles, of which there are many. One excellent article is Fluoridation/fluoride: Toxic Chemical in Your Water.

Even medications that can be life-savers can become toxic when overused or used inappropriately. Antibiotics were a fantastic discovery that protected us from diseases that were the scourge of previous ages such as syphilis, gonorrhea, pneumonia, and gangrene from wounds to name but a few. The over-prescription of antibiotics for viral and bacterial infections has led to bacteria resistance. The medical community knows perfectly well that antibiotics are ineffective against viral infections, but the public demands them and busy doctors don't have the time to argue. Though the AMA has been warning about over-prescribing antibiotics for a long time, this practice continues to the point where children have died from a scratch due to Methicillin-resistant Staphylococcus aureus (MRSA). There is also a probable association between antibiotic quantity and the cumulative number of days used and breast cancer (Emergency Medicine, November 2004). Only a few hundred women were involved in this study and more studies are needed, but surely the evidence so far indicates caution in the prescription of antibiotics.

Stress can be the result of pressure—in school, college, on the job—to perform a certain way or within a certain amount of time. All the miraculous tools that are supposed to make our lives easier have had the effect of speeding everything up. Are you of the generation that can still remember when we used to write letters, and could look forward to a couple of weeks' respite before we got an answer that we had to deal with? Now we get an email response within moments of sending a message. Our culture conditions us to expect relationships to be a certain way, and when they are not, we feel betrayed or somehow at fault. We are bombarded by a highly creative advertising industry that uses state of the art manipulation to persuade us to buy, buy, buy, which can lead to financial pressures. The sources of stress in the modern world are legion.

How does all this relate to emotional vampires? An obvious emotional vampire is someone who leeches on to you, a needy person who saps your energy. This behavior is most often unconscious, but its effect is very real. Are you aware of someone in your life that drains you? Have you ever felt suddenly tired on entering a room, or developed a headache after going into a crowded store?

Sensitive people can take on the emotional energy around them and, for example, be drained by a total stranger who passes by who is worrying about paying the grocery bill.

The vampire effect does not always have to be one individual attacking another. All of these elements discussed above—confusing childhood messages, environmental toxins, pace of life—are the vampires that drain our energy by subjecting us to stress. There are vampire organizations—and I would include the medical-pharmaceutical alliance—that have a direct negative effect on our hormonal well-being.

We have all developed ways of coping with stress, and, again, what works is very individual. Some people find a sport to be a good stress reducer, or taking a walk, a hot bath, reading, relaxing with friends, or changing the environment for a couple of days. Very often, though, we develop negative coping patterns, such as drugs, legal and illicit; alcohol; smoking; overeating; watching too much television; overspending; excessive exercise. These may soothe temporarily, but in the long term just become another source of stress.

The stress response is a hormone-driven response that involves almost all the organs of the body, and the consequences of chronic stress include hormonal imbalances that create or contribute to emotional, psychological and physical dis-ease. After 40 years of medicine and thousands of patients I am convinced that though genetics may be a predisposition for some people, in the majority of cases the pathology would stay dormant and not become overt unless stress caused it to surface. I had a personal experience that was proof enough.

A few years ago I suddenly developed a blinding headache that was unlike any pain I ever experienced before. Like the next doctor, I am my own worst patient and treated myself with everything I knew until the pain got so bad I could hardly move and could not continue to fight my wife. She took me to the emergency department where I had a CAT scan and MRI that revealed intracranial bleeding.

Ten days later I experienced severe pain in my lower right chest. Over the next six weeks I was in and out of the hospital and intensive care as a team of eight specialists tried to figure out what was going on. Finally, my hematologist Dr. Steven Mamus discovered that I have a genetic blood disorder, and the cardiologist Dr. Clayton Bredlau determined that I have a foramen ovalis, a tiny hole in my heart. By that time I had thrown numerous clots that damaged several organs.

I lived over sixty years with both of these conditions and could live many more without ever knowing anything about them. I firmly believe it was the excessive stress of the previous three or four years, on top of the cumulative stress of the decades before that, that triggered the until then dormant blood disorder gene.

Having learned the hard way, I am now practicing what I have been preaching. My hope is that I can help persuade others to begin taking better care of themselves before life gives them a painful wake-up call.

Though stress is an unavoidable fact of life, the good news, in fact the excellent news, is that you can reverse the process and take measures to protect and nurture yourself. It is within your power to take control of your own health and make the choices that will allow you to live a fuller, happier and healthier life. Our detailed program is in the final chapter but here is a simple stress reducer that you can practice anywhere, any time, even right now as you read.

The easiest and most effective way of counteracting the negative effects of stress is to learn to breathe properly and practice the complete breath regularly. If you have ever watched a baby breathe you will have noticed that the chest hardly moves at all. It is the little abdomen that inflates and deflates with the breath. At that age we all breathed the natural and healthy way, then we learned we were supposed to hold the stomach in and developed a shallow way of breathing only in to the upper chest.

Chest breathing does not fill the lower portion of the lungs with air; it is inefficient and requires more work than slow, deep, diaphragmatic breathing to accomplish the same blood/gas mixing. More work means more oxygen is needed, requiring more frequent breaths, and more blood needs to circulate through the lungs which means the heart has to work harder.

Diaphragmatic breathing means the breath is drawn all the way down into the lower lungs. If this is a new way of breathing for you it is easiest to practice lying down. Place your right hand on your chest and your left on your abdomen, and breathe the way you normally breathe and notice which hand moves. If it is only or primarily your right hand that moves, you are breathing only into the upper part of your lungs. Next concentrate on drawing the breath all the way down into your lower lungs, so that the abdomen expands on the inbreath, and deflates on the outbreath. Nothing more than that, for now.

Practice this breathing pattern for five minutes, several times a day. You can do it when you're stuck in traffic, or kept on hold. Do it when you snuggle down between the sheets at night.

Shifting from upper chest breathing to abdominal breathing is a stress reducer all by itself. But you don't have to take my word for it. Try it for a few days and see for yourself. What have you got to lose?

CHAPTER 2

Cortisol: the stress hormone

CORTISOL IS THE HORMONE THAT powers the stress response. When the body perceives a stressor, the brain signals the adrenal glands to increase the production of cortisol, which, in turn, signals all the body's systems involved in the stress response to go into high gear.

In stressful situations, the adrenal glands produce cortisol, which then stimulates the liver to put out sugar, or glucose, so that our cells can have more energy (see Appendix I). To get the influx of glucose into the cells, the pancreas is stimulated by the sugar in the blood to put out insulin, which pushes the glucose into the cells. Think of insulin as a "gatekeeper" that opens the doors in cells, allowing the sugar to come inside and be used for energy. The increased sugar and insulin is great for short-term stress, but if the stress is continuous and constant, the cycle of cortisol-liver-sugar-pancreas-insulin is continuous, which eventually causes the following problems:

Cell receptors, the part of the cell that the glucose and insulin latch on to, become fatigued from the constant stimulation of increased glucose and insulin. The result is insulin resistance, which means that the body's cells can no longer utilize the glucose for energy.

The pancreas, because it has been working overtime to produce more insulin, wears out, just like an engine wears out from constant use over time.

When the pancreas produces less insulin and the body is in a state of insulin resistance, there is more glucose in our body's blood stream instead of inside the cells where it is meant to be. This is called high blood sugar, a hallmark of Type II Diabetes.

Like the pancreas, the adrenal glands become worn out from the constant production of cortisol, known as adrenal fatigue. Do not worry about the details of this right now, it will all be explained simply and in greater detail in chapters to come.

Continuous Stress
Cortisol Reaction
(Adrenal Gland) & Effects

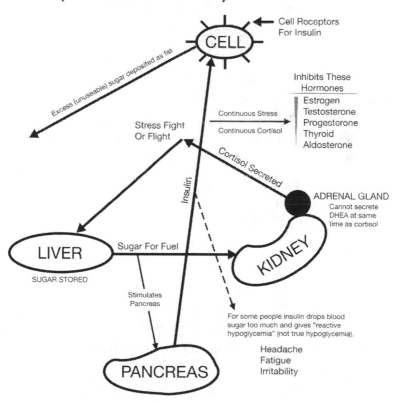

As we saw in Chapter 1, the brain reacts to mental stress the same way it reacts to physical stress. Under any kind of stress, physical, emotional or mental, the brain stimulates the stress response and releases the stress hormones; it does not differentiate between types of stress. You probably would expect your brain to know that the fight or flight response is not helpful when faced with an overbearing boss, a recalcitrant teenager, or worries about paying the mortgage—but it doesn't. The stress response can be triggered by these sorts of events or by thoughts of worry or frightening images, whether imaginary or on a movie screen.

The language of imagery is the natural language of the subconscious mind—the language of dreams, memories, and how our subconscious communicates with us. We use imagery all the time, whenever we remember an event from the past or create plans for the future. Athletes use imagery in training because, just as the stress response is triggered in response to a mental image, so the body will respond to images of performing the perfect serve or the perfect golf swing. It's as if the body does not know the difference between what we imagine happening, and what happens in the three dimensional world. The brain will stimulate the production of the same hormones to build muscle whether the athlete is visualizing or actually performing the physical act. Of course, the athlete must also physically practice so the muscles and the mind will remember what the intended action is.

We use the language of imagery all the time; most of us use the language of imagery unconsciously, and often in negative ways such as when we worry, for example. Worrying is nothing more than negative imagery—imagery that can have the power to keep us awake at night and give us tension headaches or digestive problems. These are the obvious consequences of stress, though as we proceed we will see that there are many other, not so obvious, consequences to chronic stress.

Just like athletes, all of us can learn to use imagery in positive ways—harnessing the immense power of the mind to work for us instead of against us. Many of us, for example, unconsciously absorb negative energy from our environment. Have you ever noticed that when you leave a crowded place, such as a grocery store, you feel depleted and tired? You just spent time in an environment where people tend to be rushed or may be worrying about how they are going to pay for their groceries. If you are at all sensitive you can pick up these vibrations. Imagery can be a powerful and effective way to protect ourselves from absorbing the negative emotional energy of those around us.

I discovered that caretakers were particularly susceptible to absorbing the worry energy of their charges. Often, they were taught to react in a certain way, i.e., they were "supposed" to put others' needs before their own yet they were never taught how to provide themselves with mental and physical protection. In the old days, people protected themselves from vampires with garlic; we need to learn to draw boundaries to protect ourselves from conscious and unconscious emotional vampires. All sources of stress in our lives, overt and covert, conscious and unconscious, real and imagined, trigger the stress response, which is powered by increased levels of the hormone cortisol.

During "normal," non stress-filled times, cortisol production follows a certain pattern. It is produced by the adrenal gland and is usually highest between seven and ten in the morning, though this may vary slightly depending on genetics and the time one rises. In the morning, cortisol helps awaken us by stimulating an energy burst of glucose, or sugar. This is a temporary response and throughout the day the adrenals put out steadily decreasing levels of cortisol, with the exception of a time right after meals where spurts of cortisol help the body use the carbohydrates and sugars just eaten. So, by noon the body's level of cortisol has dropped, and by six pm it is even lower. By twelve midnight it is really low, and then by five or six in the morning it starts to build up again in the blood stream. As you will see further on this diurnal cortisol flow is the reason I prefer the sputum test that gives us all four of these variations when testing for adrenal fatigue. Doing a one time blood cortisol test is not a good test.

Cortisol has many important functions in the smooth operation of the body besides powering the stress response. Cortisol is responsible for reducing inflammation; it helps thyroid hormones function properly; it helps in the metabolism of carbohydrates in conjunction with insulin; it helps to control weight; it regulates white blood cells and red blood cells. It stimulates the aromatase enzyme which converts testosterone in the fat cells to estrogen; it protects cells from excess insulin; it helps to convert fats to fatty acids and protein to amino acids so that these can be used either for sugar—for energy—or stored as glycogen in the liver for future energy needs; and it protects cells from excess insulin.

When we are under stress the natural pattern of cortisol production is disturbed. The degree of disturbance depends on the degree of stress and its duration. Because the stress response is directed towards saving the life of the organism, it takes precedence over all other functions. When cortisol is primarily focused on the stress response it is not available for all its other functions.

When a person is stressed, regardless of the source—a saber toothed tiger or a demanding mother-in-law—the body's response is the same: the fight or flight response. Adrenaline and cortisol shoot out of the adrenal gland and create the physiological responses that will help us to escape or fight. This is supposed to be short term, giving us enough time to fight or run. If the stressor is a tiger and the person escapes, the burst of physical activity signals the body to return to normal, and the adrenal's release of adrenaline and cortisol is curtailed. If the person doesn't escape and the tiger catches him, he won't have to worry about stress any more.

If, on the other hand, the stressor is the mother-in-law, the boss, or the kids, the body never gets the message to slow down. When stress is a chronic state and the adrenal gland continues to excrete cortisol we could potentially move into a pathological state. The cortisol stays high all the time, stimulating the liver to put out sugar (from its glycogen stores) for fuel so we can fight or flee. The high sugar levels stimulate the pancreas to constantly put out insulin, needed to push the sugar into the cells.

In the pursuing tiger scenario, the body uses the sugar to fuel its fight or flee response; but in the chronic stress scenario the cell cannot use all the sugar that the cortisol-liver-insulin axis delivers, so it stores the excess sugar as fat. This fat gets deposited in women in the thighs and buttocks and then the abdomen. In men it is usually deposited in the abdomen first.

Some people can experience what is called reactive hypoglycemia, which is a drastic drop in blood sugar to below the normal physiologic level that results from a surge of insulin. The blood sugar drop results in symptoms such as lethargy, angry or aggressive feelings, and they may feel sleepy. Of course, hypoglycemia stresses the body, on top of already ongoing stress. If stress continues to stimulate these reactions, eventually the receptors of the cells get tired of being hit with cortisol and become more and more resistant to the insulin. So the pancreas puts out more insulin to push the needed sugar into the cells. This vicious cycle continues causing more cell receptor resistance known as Insulin Resistance. This is the first step to diabetes mellitus (Diabetes II) and the Metabolic Syndrome (once called Syndrome X). These will be discussed in more detail in chapter 7.

The constant outpouring of cortisol can lead to other problems. One is osteoporosis. High night cortisol levels cause bone breakdown. It is for this reason that there is a warning on corticosteroid medications—synthetic pharmaceuticals that imitate natural cortisol (e.g. Prednisone)—that high cortisol levels can cause osteoporosis. Just an added aside since I mentioned the word "osteoporosis."

All of us, patients and doctors, have been conditioned to choose a medical solution rather than a lifestyle modification; this has been the increasingly dominant pattern for the past couple of generations, and so the treatment for osteopenia or osteoporosis is usually a prescription for calcium, vitamin D, sometimes synthetic hormones, or even the long-term raloxifene HCL (Evista). This is a selective estrogen receptor modulator (SERM) that prevents further bone breakdown.

However, if a SERM is taken for more than one year it lowers the levels of cortisol and DHEA (discussed later in this chapter), and blunts the adrenal cortisol response to its stimulus ACTH (adrenal corticotrophin hormone). ACTH, created by the pituitary gland, is the stimulating hormone for the adrenals to put out cortisol, especially under stress. When it is blocked and cannot do this, the adrenals will eventually atrophy and the secretions from the adrenals will cease. Therefore no cortisol and no DHEA (Genazzani, 2003). Another drug known to stop and cure osteoporosis is called Fosamax. Unfortunately some people developed osteonecrosis of the jaw, or death of the jaw bone itself, from this drug.

I believe it would be advantageous to consider the stress factor and order a sputum cortisol-DHEA test before prescribing medications. In fact, I would recommend ordering this test for all people with osteoporosis along with the other necessary lab work.

If there is no intervention to alleviate the stress situation, eventually more breakdowns in the body occur. First, the pancreas cannot keep putting out insulin constantly so it runs dry and one has full-blown diabetes II. Similarly, the adrenal gland cannot keep putting out cortisol and it runs dry, so no more cortisol. Under chronic stress conditions, first the adrenal gland overproduces cortisol, and cortisol levels are higher than normal, and then over time as the adrenal glands become depleted cortisol levels drop below normal. While the adrenal gland is preoccupied with putting out cortisol it cannot at the same time put out DHEA (dihydroepiandrosterone) which cells need as an anabolic hormone (a positive building hormone). This hormone is also a backup for making testosterone and estrogen when the body cannot produce them due to aging or other problems.

Extrapolation from
Cortisol Stress Diagram
Leading to Diabetes Melitus II

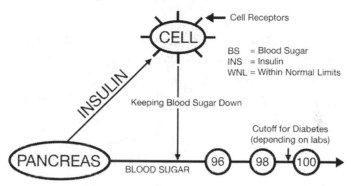

Lab reports BS 98 so physician says WNL - but if the Insulin is high it is keeping BS down. Cell receptors get tired of being hit with Insulin.

∴ Pancreas puts out more and more Insulin to compensate → Insulin Resistance
Pancreas becomes overwhelmed and stops production → Type II Diabetes

∴ Physicians need to get a fasting Insulin along with the fasting Glucose to see if the person is pre-diabetic.

Not Glucose tolerance test (GTT) but an Insulin Glucose tolerance test (IGTT) but not a plain Glucose tolerance test (GTT) to compare Insulin level to BS

∴ = Therefore

Let's look here briefly at DHEA, which will be discussed at greater length in subsequent chapters. Cholesterol makes pregnenolone. Pregnenolone is used to make DHEA or/and progesterone. The progesterone then helps make cortisol. When a vampire is attacking the body constantly the adrenal gland will put out cortisol continuously, which it would not do ordinarily. To get the building material for this quantity of cortisol the body has to steal the pregnenolone away from producing DHEA and cortisol. This is called the pregnenolone steal. In other words, when we are under stress we are taking the precursor pregnenolone—that would become DHEA—in order to make cortisol, and upsetting the balance required for efficient functioning. Our bodies need the right ratio of cortisol to DHEA for our hormonal system and immune system to function optimally. Another reason for the sputum test since it can also test the ratio between cortisol and DHEA for the diagnosis of adrenal fatigue.

These are the reasons why, when cortisol is being abnormally and constantly excreted from the adrenal gland due to stress, it is known as the death hormone. The stress response, or fight or flight response, is designed to save our lives when faced with extreme danger. To enhance this response, more of the body's resources are channeled into the systems that help us to fight or run, in order to save our lives as we saw in chapter 1: extra blood to the large muscles, extra energy to the respiratory system and circulatory systems, and so on. At the same time, energy is withdrawn from other areas that are not a priority when we are fighting for our lives, such as the digestive system and the production of certain hormones, including estrogen, testosterone, progesterone, aldosterone and thyroid.

It is this aspect of the stress response that causes imbalance and dysfunction in conditions of chronic stress. No wonder we feel terrible and become susceptible to various illnesses when under stress. All these hormones are necessary for our well-being and anti-aging. Hormone Replacement Therapy may not always help if the underlying causal factors of stress are not addressed. Patients often think that a prescribed hormone is not working, when in reality the stress is interfering with its efficacy. If the underlying cause—stress—is not addressed, it can counteract a lot of the beneficial effect of the hormone solution, whether it is one of the sex hormones or thyroid or insulin.

So often when I referred a patient to a counselor for stress management I would hear, "Please, just give me some medicine. I don't have time to eat right, or exercise, or relax." But as we have seen, all medications have side effects, and the interplay between them is highly complex and can upset the natural balance of the body. And in fact, living in the fast track, feeling guilty about taking time to relax, pushing on even during earned time-outs—by taking the computer and cell phone on vacation for example—eating processed foods and quick pick-me-ups of simple carbohydrates and coffee: the consequences of such a lifestyle cannot be fixed with medications, including hormones.

Many of us do not realize the stress we put on ourselves and the doors we open that permit emotional vampires to take advantage of us. Stress can come on unnoticed and it is often accepted and rationalized as part of our existence; this was recognized in 1936 by Hans Selye, the pioneer in stress research. Selye describes the three stages of stress, what he calls the General Adaptation Syndrome:

First, one adapts and has resistance to the stress. In this stage we may know we are pushing too hard but we accept it. Our bodies seem to be functioning fine, even though they may not feel quite like they once did.

Second, we experience adaptation to the stress, but hormones are down and we feel tired, perhaps irritable or angry, and we have symptoms that may vary according to which hormones are leading the way. The levels of some hormones may be too high while the levels of other hormones are too low.

The exhaustion stage: at this point we can no longer adapt and know we must seek medical help for continuous illness and fatigue.

In future chapters we will look at the interplay between the hormones under chronic stress conditions and will see why fixing just one is not always the solution. Because the adrenals try to adapt to chronic stress, certain hormones that would be made into other hormones (called precursors) are taken up—not to be used for their usual everyday function to keep the body in homeostasis, but rather to continue to be converted in order to "beef up" the cortisol level. Therefore, certain hormones such as progesterone and pregnenolone are detoured away from making DHEA, testosterone, estrogens and aldosterone in order to make up the depleted cortisol.

The way we react to stress controls our hormonal well-being and our health. When our mental well-being is negatively affected by people and situations that cause us stress, it affects our hormonal balance. Later we will also see how negativity, and not having an adequate support system that helps us turn negativity towards a positive way of thinking, will also affect hormonal balance.

To summarize: consistently high levels of cortisol throughout the day indicate the early stages of chronic stress. At this stage stress management procedures are highly effective. However, we have been conditioned, as a culture, to turn first to a medical solution, and to believe that there is a medication that will provide rapid relief for any symptoms. But as we know, most medications have potentially damaging side effects, and for the most part they only alleviate symptoms; they do not address the cause of discomfort or distress.

As mentioned earlier, a common response to my suggestion to learn stress management was that the patient didn't have time and just wanted medication to alleviate the uncomfortable symptoms. Many patients voiced skepticism that stress management would actually help. Is it possible that the negative response to a suggestion of lifestyle modifications would be different if there were scientific evidence proving the effectiveness of various relaxation methods in relieving stress, reducing blood pressure, and relieving tension headaches, anxiety and insomnia?

There is, in fact, extensive research on the matter, but unlike the research funded by pharmaceutical companies it is not trumpeted over the airwaves and presented in slick ads in glossy magazines. It is entombed in scholarly journals that are not readily accessible to the public. As we know, the body's response to stress is to release higher levels of cortisol. Stress levels can therefore be measured by the amount of cortisol in the saliva, urine or blood, and it is this measurement that researchers use to measure the effectiveness of natural interventions on stress levels. There are numerous studies indicating the benefits of relaxation in reducing cortisol levels and, therefore, stress levels. One of the easiest and most effective ways of achieving a state of deep relaxation is through guided imagery.

Guided imagery is a form of deliberate and directed daydreaming. It uses words and phrases that are designed to evoke a rich, multisensory fantasy that creates a state of mind receptive to desired changes in mind, body and spirit. Imagery bypasses linear thinking and logical assumptions and sends its messages directly into deep levels of the mind. Imagery is absorbed primarily through the right hemisphere of the brain by way of primitive, emotion—and sensory-based channels in the brain and nervous system. It uses the right brain's capacity for sensing, perceiving and feeling rather than the left-brain's capacity for thinking, judging, analyzing and deciding (Naparstek, 2004).

Numerous clinical trials have indicated the effectiveness of imagery in a wide variety of contexts. Many studies in the sports arena have indicated the effectiveness of imagery in training, for youth soccer players (Baron, 2000), field hockey players (Wiegardt, 1998), basketball players (Shambrook, 1996), coaching efficacy (Short, Smiley & Ross-Stewart, 2005) and dance movements (Hanrahan, 1995).

In the area of physical and mental health, the use of imagery has led to clinically significant reductions in anxiety and alteration in the illness of patients with multiple sclerosis (Maguire, 1996); contributed to general mental and physical well-being (Watanabe, Fukuda & Shirakawa, 2005); boosted the immune system (Jasnoski & Kugler, 1987); positively affected mood in healthy adults (McKinney, 1997); significantly reduced the need for opioids and hypnotics in post-surgical patients (Sohi, 1999); modulated the inflammatory response (Lutgendorf et al, 2000); and improved the quality of life in cancer patients (Burns, 2000). Conversely, guided imagery has been used as the stressor in several stress studies (Takai et al, 2004; Fox et al, 2005; Fox et al, 2006).

Guided imagery is gentle yet powerful. It is natural, self-empowering, cost-effective and free of negative side effects. The literature amply supports the effectiveness of guided imagery in creating physiological and emotional change, both in inducing the stress response—which is what we do very often in imagining negative scenarios when we worry—and in alleviating the effects of chronic stress, measured in reduced cortisol levels.

This research is easily accessible from a home computer if you are a student or an employee of a university; otherwise it requires a trip to a state university library where John Q Public is usually allowed to use any computer terminal in the reference library not required by students or faculty. There you can access the Medlit or PsychInfo databases and read the vast amount of research documenting the benefits, not only of guided imagery, but also of progressive muscle relaxation, Yoga, T'ai Chi, self hypnosis and various forms of meditation in alleviating stress, reducing blood pressure, and boosting the immune system. Check the keywords "cortisol" and "relaxation." The same keywords will also bring up studies indicating reduced blood pressure and improved immune function as a result of relaxation training.

As we have seen, the initial response to stress is high cortisol levels, but the adrenal gland cannot continue to produce cortisol constantly and indefinitely. Eventually it wears out, and cortisol levels drop. Consistently low levels of cortisol indicate the advanced stage of chronic stress, known as adrenal fatigue, and here—along with stress management—medical intervention is necessary to support the adrenals until they can recover and begin producing cortisol and DHEA again. Often, this can be accomplished with stress management and natural supplements, though in extreme cases cortisol replacement may be necessary.

The amount of time it takes to progress from high to low levels of cortisol depends on many variables: the level of stress, genetics, and the degree of emotional, mental and spiritual resources.

There are certain signs and symptoms that one should look for if low cortisol levels (adrenal fatigue) are suspected. (See Appendix III for the clinical tests for adrenal fatigue). The following are clues:

- morning fatigue: you do not awaken easily and stay groggy until about ten o'clock
- you feel awake from ten to twelve, especially after lunch
- you experience a low about two to four in the afternoon and then pick up again around six with this burst you are tired again by nine or ten, but if you stay up you get another energy burst until about one or two in the morning
- your best sleep is between seven and nine in the morning
- during the day you need a lot of caffeine to keep going
- cravings, e.g. for salt
- you hyperventilate (frequent sighing and rapid breathing)
- liver spots (chloasma)
- frequent colds and allergies
- feelings of helplessness (which cause more stress)

The best way to test cortisol levels, I believe, is through saliva testing four times a day. As we have seen, cortisol by nature changes its day-night production output. It is high in the morning, and then by noon it is dropping and by evening it is down and is even lower at midnight. It starts to go up again about five or six in the morning so that we can wake up with a sugar spurt. A blood test would only show the cortisol level at one particular time, and not give the healer the knowledge of this diurnal/nocturnal trend. Also, for some people getting stuck by a needle is stressful and can trigger the stress response, which will influence the cortisol level. Saliva testing is very simple; you collect a small amount of saliva in a glass tube at specific times of day and night, and the samples are sent to a lab for analysis.

CHAPTER 3

Cholesterol and Hormones

FOR SOME TIME THERE HAS been a big medical drive to bring down everybody's cholesterol. This lowering of the total cholesterol is driven by antiquated academics and the pharmaceutical companies' sales propaganda directed both to the public and to physicians. At one time scientists and physicians thought that cholesterol was the only cause of arteriosclerosis (hardening of the arteries), and therefore was the main reason for cardiovascular disease. This is past history and has been surpassed by new evidence, not only as to what causes cardiovascular problems, but also the importance of cholesterol and other good fats such as omega 3s.

The facts are these: It is inflammation and free radicals that deteriorate the heart and its vessels. There are marker tests that would show these inflammations, such as homocysteine, fibrinogen and C-reactive protein heart specific (CRP-hs). They are too often not ordered and insurance companies too often will not pay for them.

In any case, high cholesterol is not the villain of heart disease as most of us have been told. Even the AMA admits that 51% of heart attack patients who enter emergency rooms do not have high cholesterol. All the emphasis on lowering total cholesterol fails to take into consideration the healthy functions of cholesterol, which is their basic biochemical configuration from which the hormones cortisol, aldosterone, testosterone, progesterone, estrogen, and Vitamin D are produced. (See Appendix I for these hormones and their functions).

We have already discussed the important role of cortisol as the main stress indicator in chapter 2. Another function of the cortisol hormone is to act as an antioxidant, protecting the body by preventing oxidation from free radicals.

FREE RADICALS

"Free radical oxidation" is a term often used in the news and in health advertisements, but I have found that many of my patients don't know what it means. A "free radical" is a molecule that has an unpaired electron. Electrons should always be evenly paired, like a loving couple. When they are not in a pair they seek to steal an electron from another molecule. "Oxidation" is when these free radical molecules want to find a mate to make a pair of electrons and therefore attack other molecules to capture one of the electrons from them. This changes the chemical configuration of the attacked molecule as it then becomes a molecule with an unpaired electron. So a chain reaction starts: each unpaired molecule attacks another molecule and in the process damages the makeup of whatever tissue these molecules comprise as a structure.

Free radical damage is a bit like nano BBs constantly bombarding the endothelium, or lining, of the inner arterial walls. As it does in the case of any injury, such as a cut on the skin, the body sends out its rescue immune white blood cells and cells called fibrocytes. Fibrocytes are cells that help form scabs to protect the skin after a cut. Something similar happens when the inner arterial wall is damaged by free radicals, and over time this builds into a plaque, or atheroma, that can keep growing and narrowing or even closing off the arterial circulation at that point. It can also protrude into the lumen, or the hollow opening in the middle of a blood vessel that the blood flows through. When this happens, it is called a thrombus, which is another word for a type of clot within the blood vessels and it is much like a scab on a cut. This clot can break off and travel through the circulatory system (when a clot breaks off it is called an embolus) until it gets stuck in a smaller artery and causes a plug. The plug stops oxygen and nutrition from getting to that tissue, and we have a cardiac infarct, if it gets stuck in the heart, or a stroke, if it gets stuck in the brain.

The magic number

There is a common belief that a total cholesterol above 200 is too high and increases the danger of heart disease. Often, patients exhibiting a higher total cholesterol level are prescribed a cholesterol lowering called a "statin." It is important, however, to consider not so much the total cholesterol, as the components of that number; not all cholesterol is bad and some is really important.

Let's briefly review the components of cholesterol:

High Density Lipoproteins (HDL): good cholesterol. They are considered the good fats because they take the "bad" cholesterol (Low Density Lipoproteins or LDL) from other areas of the body, such as the arteries, and return it to the liver where it can either be eliminated—if in abundance—or used for different functions. According to Michael Murray, raising the HDL by 1% will decrease the risk of a cardiac event by 2%. The considered normal HDL value is more then 45mg/dl. If the HDL is high it is making up a big portion of the total cholesterol, which could be why your health provider is reading your total cholesterol as high. Be sure to check to the HDL to see if it is the cause of elevated total cholesterol.

Low Density Lipoproteins (LDL). The LDLs are considered bad cholesterol because this is the type of cholesterol that becomes deposited in the arteries and other organs, especially when they are in abundance and the quantity cannot be taken back to the liver by the HDL. They are the fats that are considered the cause of cardiovascular events. Just as a 1% increase in HDLs decreases the risk of a cardiac event by 2%, a 1% drop in LDLs decreases the risk of a heart attack by 2%. The considered normal value of LDL is less then 100mg/dl.

Triglycerides are the most abundant fats in the human body, and are found in such foods as seeds, yolks and animal fats. There are very few of them in vegetables. Triglycerides can be helpful or harmful depending on the concentration in our bodies and the normal level is considered to be less than 150mg/dl. They are used as body insulation since they are found just under the skin, dampening shock waves when we bump into things, and are even found in the fat pad under the heel. Mainly they are the emergency source of energy and serve as a reserve for the essential omega-3s and omega-6s.

The danger of triglycerides is when they are consumed in excess, by eating too much sugar (which in excess is converted to a large degree into triglycerides), and too much saturated fat. In this case the triglyceride is oxidized; it can damage the interior walls of the arteries, and cause red blood cells to clump together.

The Cardiac heart ratio is total cholesterol divided by HDL. This is a value that gives the physician or healer another statistic to evaluate a patient's potential for a cardiovascular event or to monitor a client who is following a regimen. There are various ways of doing this. I like to use the total cholesterol/HDL giving a value of less then 3.5 Other healers use what is called the Cardiac risk Factor which is LDL/HDL wanting a value of less then 4.5.

So you can see, the cholesterol situation is more complex than simply the number representing the total cholesterol. A high total cholesterol level of 200 plus may not be so bad if it is made up of mostly HDL cholesterol. Even if the LDLs are high, that's not so bad either if the particles making up the LDL are large particles. If the LDLs are in the normal range but are made up of small particles they are more dangerous than if they are in the high count but made up of large particles of LDL. In other words, it is the size of the LDL particle and not just the amount of the LDL noted in the lab report that is important. It is possible to measure the type of LDL, and therefore get a more accurate account of the potential risk. The types of LDL are called apolipoprotein (a) and apolipoprotein (b) and the tests are called apolipoprotein a test and apolipoprotien b test (Zubrod, 2006). The moral of the story is, cholesterol is more than just a number, and all of the factors I have just mentioned must be taken into account before prescribing a cholesterol lowering drug with potentially dangerous side effects.

As we have seen, damage to the lining of the arteries can have disastrous consequences. I mentioned that free-radicals can damage the arterial lining, but how does LDL cause damage? First, for the arteries to be affected by the LDL, there needs to be an injury that allows the LDL to enter into the inner arterial lining, or endothelium. The entry point is caused by entities such as bacteria, high levels of insulin, certain minerals or heavy metals such as mercury and cadmium, which is from cigarettes; and, of course, the free radicals as we explained above. It is not the LDL that is the initial cause, but an infiltration of the LDL after other injuries caused by such entities as were mentioned above which, over time, cause microscopic openings in the arterial wall.

LOW CHOLESTEROL

All the emphasis and fear around high cholesterol has eclipsed the dangers of low cholesterol, which are many:

A person with total cholesterol of less than 180 has a 2.7 times greater chance of being depressed. Suicide rates may also relate to this low number (Ellison & Morrison, 2001; Golier et al, 1995). It is not infrequent for a person to come to me with feeling of malaise, low libido, depression, and fatigue because their cholesterol is so low from being on statin drugs that they cannot produce sex hormones, vitamin D, cortisol and aldosterone. Low Vitamin D is also being associated with depression.

And there are other risks associated with low cholesterol. About 60% of the brain is fat, a lot of it from cholesterol. I joke around when lecturing that, when someone calls you a fat-head, you should say thank you.

Fat also forms the myelin sheath around the nerves, which protects the nerves and helps conduct incredibly fast nerve impulses, sort of like the insulation around an electric wire.

Recently there has been scientific evidence indicating that cholesterol plays a role in the synapse between nerves, the space that lets the nerve impulse jump from one nerve to the next. In people over the age of 75, some studies show the higher their cholesterol the longer they live, of course levels within reason—about 250mg/dl (Xumei Huang, 2007). This study also indicates that, "patients with low levels of LDL cholesterol are at least three and half times more likely to develop Parkinson's disease then those with higher LDL levels."

Another problem that low fats create in men is emasculation, because cholesterol is necessary for the production of testosterone. Low cholesterol may result in lower levels of testosterone, which may be the source of the man's problem, but the ally of the Viagra industry.

We all know that vitamin D is important in so many functions of our bodies, from prevention of osteoporosis to a cofactor in the problem of depression. Inadequate dietary intake of the proper fats has led to a lack of vitamin D in our western society. Statistically this is about 28.8% in women and 13.6% in men. (InChianti, 2007).

Certain vitamins—A, D, E, and K depend on dietary fat for their absorption. The New England Journal of Medicine, June 1998, had some studies on vitamin D deficiency. For those who wish to delve further into this topic there is much being studied and written about Vitamin D, which some physicians now consider a hormone.

Here, the emotional vampire is our medical/pharmaceutical consortium. The physiological stress caused by the lack of hormones and vitamins due to having the cholesterol and fats diverted from our bodies is quite obvious. There are numerous disruptive and stressful consequences that contribute to poor emotional well being, all of which can be attributed to lacking a physiological amount of good fats and cholesterol. Diminished levels of sex hormones, the fear and consequences of osteoporosis, and also effect on the family when a member commences to dementia—or any malady that the statin drugs have the potential to cause.

STATIN DRUGS

All the focus on lowering total cholesterol levels has led to high dependence on the cholesterol-lowering drugs known as statins. Now that we have seen how lowering cholesterol levels too far means that the cholesterol base is not available to make other needed substances such as hormones, lets take a closer look at this "magical" group of drugs. Statin drugs may have deleterious side effects; in fact, there is a warning in the informational insert about the dangerous effects they can have on the liver. Liver function tests (LFT's), blood tests that clinicians use to gauge the health of the liver, need to be done biannually for those taking statin drugs. But that's not the only side effect:

Statin drugs carry warnings about rhabdomyolosis, which is muscle break-down that results in muscle pain (myalgia). When this occurs, the patient should be immediately taken off the drug, but all too often they are just changed to another statin, or the diagnosis of the causal agent (the statin drug) is missed and the patient is put on a non-steroidal anti-inflammatory drug, or NSAID, for the pain. The problem is that, if the rhabdomyolosis persists, it may never be cured, even if the drug is stopped. There is a simple blood test that shows the breakdown of muscle: if the creatine metabolite (creatine kinase) in the blood is elevated, there is muscle breakdown and the statin should be stopped. Creatine kinase that is detected in the blood is a byproduct of muscle breakdown.

In Canada there is also a warning on the statin insert that statins will deplete enzyme CoQ10. This is because the same pathway the statin is using for lowering cholesterol also stops the production of CoQ10. CoQ10 is an enzyme produced by the liver and is used for making energy for muscles, including the heart muscle. CoQ10 is needed to make ATP (adenosine triphosphate), a chemical used by all cells to make energy. Without ATP we lose or depress functions because we don't have enough fuel to run the engine. Supplemental CoQ10 is necessary if statin drugs are taken but too often is not suggested to the patient.

Statin drugs have been implicated in forgetfulness, and as being one of the co-factors for either causing dementias or being an adjunct to dementia. In fact, cognitive problems are an outstanding complaint with the statin drugs. This is very likely due to the fact that the brain also needs ATP to function. It is usually a temporary condition called transient global amnesia (TGA); the patient sometimes cannot even remember their spouse. This came into view when former astronaut Duane Graveline MD was put on Lipitor and developed TGA. He wrote a book about the statins called *Lipitor, Thief of Memory*. As mentioned, this is usually a temporary condition that disappears when the drug is stopped, but whether there are other memory problems after long-term statin use has not yet been studied.

The brain depends on cholesterol, other fatty acids and ATP to be strong and function properly. When someone gets a "foggy brain" they are still alert enough to know that they are not functioning at their usual level. This leads to stress that only compounds the problem. The Framingham study disclosed that older persons with cholesterol under 200 perform worse on mental function tests than those with higher cholesterol (about 250mg/dl). Numerous articles are available both for and against this theory, but like any of our evidence-based drug studies it is necessary to be careful about who did the study and who paid for it. All too often the drug company producing the pharmaceutical supported the positive studies in one way or another, and may have suppressed any negative studies.

Women taking Lipitor, a brand-name statin drug and at one time the best-selling drug in the USA, had 10% more heart attacks then the control group taking a placebo (Whitaker, 2007).

For people over 70 years of age there is no research that there is life prolongation by taking statin drugs. The same holds true for young men with high cholesterol without heart disease: statins do not influence their longevity in any studies (ibid).

Statin drugs may have their place, but there are many natural ways to lower cholesterol safely, with botanicals, diet and exercise, and I strongly believe they should be tried first. I believe that statin drugs should have a place only in specific circumstances and usually after a change of lifestyle is programmed and followed for at least 6-12 months.

If statins are used the patient should be followed closely for any signs or symptoms of side effects. The drug should also be stopped when the total cholesterol falls below 160-170, because a sufficient amount of cholesterol is essential for our well-being.

I have found that relying on medications often gives the patient the impression that they can continue to follow an unhealthy lifestyle as long as they are on medication. As you no doubt know, quite apart from the dangers of side effects, medications are all too often just alleviating symptoms while the cause remains unaddressed. I have had many patients who presented with high blood pressure, for instance, for which they were often taking medication. Most often after a ten minute hypnosis session the blood pressure came down, indicating that stress was causing the problem and that daily relaxation would alleviate it without the need for drugs. In the same way, high levels of LDLs can often be brought back down to acceptable levels through diet, exercise and stress management. LDLs may respond to regimens of supplements recommended by an informed holistic physician.

For our primary purpose here, the important thing to remember is that cholesterol is necessary for the production of essential hormones: cortisol, aldosterone, testosterone, progesterone, estrogen and vitamin

D, which many researchers consider a hormone. When cholesterol levels are too low, production of all these necessary components of good health are compromised.

The use of Statin drugs may not be appropriate for everyone and there should be careful patient selection based upon who will achieve the most benefit. This is not only my view, but it is due to the many possible side effects such as: muscle pain and deterioration (rhabdomyolosis) fatigue, memory loss (transient global amnesia =TGA), liver problems, and the FDA reports that diabetes could also be a real side effect.

In his book, *The Creative Destruction of Medicine*, author and chief academic officer of Scripps Health, Eric Topol writes, "One or two out of 100 patients without prior heart disease but at risk for developing such a condition will actually benefit, but how about the 98 out of 100?" Also note that the Scandinavian Simvastatin Survival Study (a statin drug) showed that treating patients with pre-existing heart disease decreased their chance of dying over five years from 12 percent, without statin drugs, to 8 percent with statin drugs. So, if you were in the pre-existing heart attack class, you would probably want to take the statins but also with the awareness of the possible side effects. So what Eric Topol is saying, is that the statins can reduce your possibility of a cardiovascular event by about 2-4%; not really significant, but worth considering before deciding whether to take statins or not.

NNT stands for "Number Needed to Treat," which is to show what a drug can do for the quantity of people taking it to help them. For example, sixty people would need to take a statin drug for five years for one person to avoid a heart attack. The NNT for a stroke prevention with a statin, if 268 people took them over five years, only one person would not have a stroke. These NNT statistics are from the Mount Sinai Medical Center in New York by Dr. David

Newman. Dr Newman also states that, "Cholesterol levels are not as strongly predictive of cardiovascular disease as once thought. This has shocked everyone. Cholesterol levels are actually a fairly weak predictor of who will have a heart attack." I must state that I have not found his original article and apologize for this, even if I do agree that inflammation to the cardiovascular system is the more concerning factor for cardiovascular disease.

This last part of the statin drug portion of this book was reported in the Saturday Evening Post, not a scientific journal, but by well-known author Sharon Begley who wrote *The Emotional Life of Your Brain.*

As stated already, one does have to consider risk verses benefit and make a choice with your physician. For example: Five percent of people on statins will develop rhabdomyolysis (muscle pain and breakdown). The New York Times in 2012 stated that taking statins makes it harder to exercise, which could possibly be due to muscle breakdown. Also, there is the possibility that this drug makes the body's repair of muscle damage more difficult.

The Mayo Clinic reported in The Archives of Internal Medicine that the use of statins in postmenopausal women increased their risk of new-onset diabetes to 71 %.

In February, the FDA mandated labeling on statins warning people that statins can cause certain cognitive problems like memory loss (TGA=Transient Global Amnesia). The FDA also mandates labeling to include a warning about increased risk of Type II Diabetes.

As an holistic physician I still believe the choice is to discuss all options and pros and cons with your personal physician. Some may need the statins and others may not. Some may need to change their life style only and need neither pharmaceuticals nor supplements. One thing is clear—we must give intellectual thought to medications and supplements without rationalization and prejudice.

CHAPTER 4

Hormones and Their Functions

I AM GOING TO APPROACH each individual hormone in a way that is slightly different from just enumerating their effects on the body, which can be found in any endocrinology or medical physiology book (and also in Appendix II). I hope to show the importance of each individual hormone and it's relationship to the topic of illness due to the vampire effect.

Let's begin by reiterating the connection between cortisol and stress; as mentioned, when cortisol levels are consistently high it is known as the "death hormone" because greater and more continuous quantities than nature planned can have deleterious effects, as we saw in the last chapter until the adrenals collapse and produce little to no cortisol, which is called adrenal fatigue.

For the purposes of the present discussion, we need to remember that elevated levels of cortisol as a result of stress lower the quantity of other hormones: testosterone, aldosterone, estrogen, progesterone, and thyroid, because they are not needed for the fight or flight response in perceived situations of life or death.

I'd like to start with the misunderstood hormone testosterone, which has gotten the reputation of just being a male hormone to annoy women. This is not true! In both males and females there are 3-4 times more testosterone cell receptors in the heart than in the sex glands. Testosterone also helps to create more nitric oxide, a substance which dilates, or opens, blood vessels. This last affect is similar to the use of nitroglycerin for angina and chest pain. Therefore, testosterone protects the heart, otherwise Nature would not have provided these functions for testosterone.

As for the brain, low levels of testosterone can cause slower thinking and when it gets too low one cannot even fantasize. These last two effects of testosterone were found using an fMRI (functional magnetic resonance imaging), an MRI that shows what part of the brain is being used for different functions. Newer studies show that low testosterone in males may be directly related to a higher incidence of Alzheimer's disease. In fact, in one study synthetic testosterone was administered to Alzheimer patients; it did not cure them but it did significantly slow down the progression of the disease (Resnick & Moffat, 2007; Pike et al, 2006).

It is well known that testosterone builds muscle. If you work out in a gym, you may have noticed that as men get older, no matter how intense their workouts, they will still get flabby, especially the pectoral or chest muscles. This will occur if they do not take supplemental testosterone to compensate for their declining production of this hormone. Compare this to building a really nice house. If the foundation is not strong and built with the right materials the house will not be stand.

There are other important jobs for this hormone. Testosterone is important in preventing osteoporosis and osteopenia, which are diseases where the bones become thin and brittle. Look at it this way: men do not get osteoporosis usually until their late sixties or older, whereas in women it can begin as early as mid forties. Why? Because men have thick bones from having larger amounts of testosterone than women throughout their youth. Testosterone is the real bone-building hormone in both men and women.

To be sure, progesterone helps build bones by way of promoting cells called osteoblasts, (which build bone), and yes, as John Lee M.D. states, estrogen helps prevent osteoporosis by preventing the reabsorption of bone by osteoclasts, (which break down bone), but the decline in testosterone levels during perimenopause or menopause also contributes to osteoporosis because testosterone is the big bone builder. That is why men do not get osteopenia or osteoporosis until they are much older than women, if at all. I have given women patients small amounts of natural testosterone, not synthetic pharmaceuticals, for osteoporosis and osteopenia with beneficial results. Those who begin taking testosterone at perimenopause do not acquire osteoporosis or osteopenia. So, as far as anti-aging goes, for men and women to keep muscle tone and bone stability testosterone replacement at physiological dosages should be discussed with a knowledgeable physician.

A note about hormone replacement therapy (HRT): Like any other hormone deficiency, deficient testosterone in men and women will interfere with a healthy and vigorous life and contribute to aging. It can easily be remedied by taking testosterone, but, unfortunately, this remedy is often avoided because of misunderstandings and myths about the role of testosterone.

Testosterone earned a bad reputation from publicity resulting from its abuse by athletes. However, there are two important points to bear in mind regarding testosterone abuse by athletes. First of all, they were using synthetic testosterone and the body does not know what to do with synthetic chemicals that have molecular structures that are different from those produced naturally by the body. For therapeutic purposes I would recommend only bio-identical testosterone, meaning testosterone that has the same molecular structure as that produced naturally by the body.

Secondly, when athletes abuse testosterone, it is used in enormous quantities. As with any medication, natural or pharmaceutical, the dose must be appropriate and individualized to the person. Many athletes were taking enormous doses in order to artificially boost their muscle mass and their athletic performance, not what would be an appropriate dose to bring their testosterone to a normal level.

Note again that when I talk about HRT, I am talking about bio-identical hormones, hormones that have the same molecular structure as those produced naturally by the body, not synthetic hormones that have a slightly different molecular structure. Pharmaceutical companies, because of the differences in molecular structure, can patent synthetic hormones whereas bio-identical hormones are not patented.

Brad was a 57-year-old male who sat down on the other side of my desk looking bewildered and apprehensive. He had the face of a man who wanted to talk but did not know how to begin. "Okay, Dr. Sault," he finally said, "I have a problem with getting fatigued easily. Actually, I don't have any energy at all. And my concentration is shot. I used to be full of energy and had a lot of incentive to do my job, but now I feel like I can barely get out of bed."

I asked Brad if he exercised regularly. "Sure, always have. I work out 3-4 times a week with weights and the other days I run. I've always been in good shape but now, just look at me. I've got this big belly and I'm even . . . I'm even getting flabby up here." And indeed through his T-shirt I could see that Brad had developed flabby breasts. "And even though it sounds crazy, I know I'm getting shorter! And round shouldered."

"What about your mood?"

He shook his head. "My wife tells me I act depressed and quite irritable. I know she's right but I don't seem to be able to help it."

"And what about your sex drive?"

He looked very uncomfortable. "To be honest, doc, I'm not that interested. And when I am I have a hard time getting it up, or keeping it up. I feel inadequate. I think my wife thinks there's something wrong with our relationship but I just can't bring myself to discuss this with her. And, as long as I'm being so frank, I also have a problem peeing. I have to go pretty often, especially at night, and it just takes forever. It comes out in a weak, slow stream."

In women, production of the sex hormones estrogen and progesterone falls quite suddenly usually between the ages of 50 and 58, leading to the well-known symptoms of menopause. In men, production of testosterone begins to decline at around age 35, but the decline is so slow that the effects are not usually felt until around Brad's age, when low testosterone causes his presenting symptoms and the stage of life known as "andropause," often referred to as "mens' menopause." See Appendix IV for a comparison of the signs and symptoms of menopause and andropause.

Many men fear taking bio-identical testosterone to counteract the symptoms of andropause, partly because of the reasons given above, and partly because of the old myth that testosterone will cause prostate cancer. This has been disproved and, in fact, the guilty hormone is estrogen. A recent article on a study conducted in Korea shows that men with low testosterone are more likely to get prostate cancer than men with higher testosterone levels. This was a study involving 568 men using both prostate biopsy and following along with PSA (Prostate Specific Anti body) tests. (Shin, Hwang et al., *Is a Decreased Serum Testosterone Level a Risk Factor for Prostate Cancer? A Cohort Study of Korean Men* Dec 5, 2010 1(12:819-23)

All fetuses start as a female and during fetal development the genes will kick in to trigger the transition to a male fetus. There remains, inside the prostate, a remnant of the would-be uterus called a utricle. It is this little villain that gets hit with estrogen to cause cancer of the prostate. Whether testosterone will cause an existing cancer to grow faster is still to be determined, but so far the evidence is against this. There is another prevalent myth regarding testosterone—that it causes clotting. In fact, not only does testosterone not cause clotting, it actually prevents it (Smith et al, 2005).

If the patient and doctor decide that testosterone replacement is to be done, I recommend the following tests to be performed beforehand:

1. A male must have blood tests for his estrogen levels and PSA levels (prostate specific antigen) to be safe. Since testosterone can convert to estrogen it is wise to know what the levels are before therapy and about 3-6 months after therapy commences.
2. Complete blood count (CBC).

3. I also like a base line of liver functions. The liver rids the body of excess estrogen and if the liver is not functioning properly the excess estrogen is not eliminated as it should be.

4. There is always the possibility that testosterone will convert to estrogen, especially in the presence of synthetic hormones or too much testosterone. This phenomenon is called aromatization because the aromatase enzyme, which is found in the fat cells, causes it. It is easy to test for this by ordering tests of estradiol levels; if this level is increased, the person is aromatizing.

5. DHT (dihydrotestosterone) levels should be tested if the patient believes he is going bald or has an enlarged prostate. The baldness may be genetic and the prostate may be enlarging as can happen to men as they get older. But, in order to be sure, it is best to see if testosterone is converting to too much DHT, since there are things the physician can do to alleviate this conversion. I do this after the client is on testosterone and having signs of conversion to DHT.

6. I order a test of total testosterone, which is just that, the total amount of testosterone in the body. I will also test for what is called free testosterone because this test measures the amount of testosterone that can be used by the body's cells. It does not matter if the total testosterone is good if there is not enough free testosterone to enter the cells and do the work. To understand what free testosterone is, you must know that hormones can be attached to, or "bound," to proteins. When a hormone is bound up it is made useless, but if the hormone is "free" it is not attached to a protein and, therefore, is readily available to be used by the body's cells. The proteins that bind to hormones originally, through evolution, developed to protect from an overload of certain hormones. I will test for the binding proteins, specifically one called SHBG (sex hormone binding globulin) that can bind up the testosterone and render it useless to the cells. SHBG is

a protein hormone that is capable of binding testosterone, and some people genetically produce a lot more then necessary.

The physician may order different tests for different patients, based on the interview and physical and the patient's specific needs.

See Appendix V for a full list of recommended tests for men and women before and during HRT.

Once again, I must return to the topic of stress. If the testosterone is too high, then cortisol falls. But if cortisol is elevated due to stress, then testosterone goes down. Cortisol, as already mentioned, evolved as a "fight or flight" protection. Therefore, certain hormones that are not needed for this short burst of activity are inhibited by the cortisol. Testosterone is one of them.

Those people who are receiving human identical hormones and still not getting beneficial results may believe that the physician is not adjusting the hormones properly. This is possible, but do not dismiss the very strong probability that the underlying cause may be stress or another ailment. The emotional state can affect the hormonal balance. In other words, a person who is depressed or taking on more then they can physically and /or mentally handle will not magically feel great due to hormonal correction alone; the underlying emotional detour needs to be fixed. For optimal health, all the hormones have to be in balance with one another and we now know that stress can upset this balance.

For example, the male who cannot get an erection and believes that testosterone is the answer may remain in the same deflated state if there is an emotional issue between him and his partner(s). In this case a Viagra-like drug may alleviate his erectile dysfunction but it will not cure the problem. Without going for the cure, the underlying problem is going to affect his erection and probably more aspects of his life and health, besides the potential deleterious side effects of Viagra and its cousin. I could write a book of examples of clients, both men and women, who believed that HRT therapy did not fix all "my life's problems" because they were not willing to solve the real emotional-spiritual problems underlying their hormonal imbalance. The hormones can be balanced by the physician but the mind has to be balanced as well and this requires the participation of the client.

If you refer to the chart (Appendix IV) comparing Menopause and Andropause, you will see that Brad had a deficiency of testosterone. He also had a prostate problem because of his urinary symptoms. The urinary problem had to be explored further to rule out cancer, although these kinds of symptoms are usually benign prostate hypertrophy (BPH), or harmless enlargement of the prostate gland. Counseling for any psychological and marital problems that had arisen during his uncorrected testosterone problem was also recommended.

Aldosterone is a hormone that is probably not familiar to most of my readers. It controls the sodium-potassium also known as electrolytes balance in the body. Sodium and potassium are minerals that are also referred to as electrolytes and are partially responsible for maintaining blood pressure and other cellular functions. Aldosterone is a hormone that is affected by cortisol and therefore can be influenced by stress.

Aldosterone, like cortisol, is produced in the adrenal glands, a small gland that is situated on top of each kidney, and follows a diurnal pattern, as does cortisol. Remember that a 'diurnal pattern' means that hormone levels follow a pattern of release during the 24 hour day.

In response to stress, the pituitary gland, located in the head near the brain, produces more ACTH (adrenocorticotrophic hormone). This stimulates cortisol production, and aldosterone just tags along with this stimulus. Aldosterone also peaks with cortisol under stress. In other words, it is increased during stress. However, after 24 hours of output the adrenal gland can no longer manufacture aldosterone, even if the body needs it for its physiological functions.

It is persistent, elevated levels of aldosterone, as described above, that leads in part to the symptoms and signs of adrenal fatigue. As mentioned, aldosterone controls the sodium-potassium balance in our bodies, and therefore has a major role in regulating blood pressure, since these two minerals play a major role in blood pressure control. A high concentration of aldosterone will increase sodium and at the same time decrease potassium. The opposite is also true; lack of aldosterone will cause a loss of sodium and an increase of potassium, this will be seen in the lack of sodium in the urine. An increase of sodium causes the body to compensate by having a greater absorption of water. This, in turn, will increase the blood pressure. The feedback to the kidneys causes the kidneys to excrete more salt and water. As long as the aldosterone stays high so will the blood pressure. Meanwhile, the potassium is falling. It is the sodium-potassium balance that the nerve cells and muscle cells of the body (including the heart) depend on for their electrical stimulation and proper function. Other electrolytes are required as well, but here we are primarily concerned with sodium and potassium.

The sodium chloride/potassium-magnesium homeostasis is what maintains the electrical capacities in our muscles and nerves. It is what keeps the proper amount of fluid in the blood and in the interstitial fluids (the fluids between the cells) and the intrastitial fluids (the fluids in our cells). These minerals, or electrolytes, are responsible for the efficient functioning of our nerve and muscle cells. They are usually tested for when a physician does a comprehensive blood analysis for your physical.

If aldosterone is deficient, the potassium concentrations will rise, which can cause cardiac toxicity in the way of cardiac muscle weakness. This means the heart has weak contractions, and can lead to dysrhythmias, or an irregular heartbeat, and eventually heart failure and death.

As we certainly know by now, during stress cortisol levels rise. Because the human animal wants above all to survive, the built-in protective mechanisms of the stress response use the higher cortisol levels to make the body a more efficient fighting or running machine. In the process, it lowers the production of anything that is not pertinent to the cause, including unneeded hormones such as aldosterone (along with thyroid, testosterone, estrogen and progesterone); unneeded, of course, in the restricted context of fighting or fleeing, which is supposed to last only a short time. When you've won the fight or fled to a safe distance, the body is supposed to return to normal. In the case of chronic stress, the protracted lowering of aldosterone causes a loss of sodium and elevation of potassium, and eventually causes the muscles and nerves to fire improperly. They become fatigued, as does the heart and the person in general.

The loss of sodium and therefore fluids with it would make the blood pressure too low. The lowering of aldosterone also makes the kidneys excrete more sodium, and it takes water with it. To compensate for this water loss the body pulls the interstitial and intrastitial fluids into the blood stream to try to keep a good blood volume. As this intrastitial water is pulled from the cells it is taking sodium out of the cells and the cells themselves become dehydrated. Because the cells have to have the right ratio of sodium to potassium, the potassium also is eventually pulled out of the cells. Therefore, it is quite possible that a blood test will show the electrolytes to be normal, because of this compensation: the cells giving up their electrolytes to the blood stream to maintain the sodium/potassium ratio within the cells. But in actuality the cells are becoming depleted of their electrolytes or/and becoming dehydrated, since water follows sodium out of the cells. The effect of this cellular dehydration is fatigue of body and mind.

Now we are going to get into the more familiar female hormones; remember, however, that both males and females have the same hormones but in different quantities and ratios. Sometimes the symptoms of excess and deficiency are similar in both sexes, and sometimes different. In this section we will be addressing the two predominant female hormones: estrogen and progesterone, but it is important to know that testosterone is important to the female well-being.

Let me say again that when I talk about hormone replacement therapy (HRT) I refer only to the bio-identical hormones that are chemically identical to the hormones produced by the body. I actually prefer the term "human bio-identical hormones."

The media hysteria as a result of the discontinuation of the Women's Health Initiative Study has created much confusion and much fear around HRT. In case you missed it, the 2002 WHIS followed 166,8080 women using synthetic estrogen and progestin, a synthetic progesterone, which is not a true progesterone. The study was stopped early because of higher than average illnesses among the subjects. These included coronary heart disease (29%), stroke (41%), venous thromboembolism (blood clots: 11%), breast cancer (26%), colorectal cancer (37%) and hip fracture (34%) (Journal of the American Medical Association, 2002.)

However, the subjects of this study were receiving synthetic hormones, which have a slightly different molecular configuration from those naturally produced by the body. Pharmaceutical companies can patent synthetic hormones; one cannot patent natural substances. The body treats synthetics as foreign substances and just is not sure how to react to them in a fully positive way. So, in the case of synthetic hormones, there are some positive stimuli and some very serious deleterious effects as seen by the WHI study. Note that the progestin used in the study is a synthetic pharmaceutical hormone and is not nature's progesterone.

Natalie presented as a well-dressed, sophisticated business woman. She was 47 years old and married with two grown children who did not live at home. Her major complaint was fatigue, present for about one year and becoming more and more "burdensome." She was also gaining weight though she exercised regularly with both resistance and cardiovascular workouts. She noticed that it was taking her a longer time to recover after exercising. She began experiencing frequent headaches—a new experience for her. Her tolerance for her family and colleagues was volatile. She believes that this decreased tolerance was due to fatigue and the headaches she suffered frequently.

She had been married for 22 years but no longer had much of a libido and she believed her husband thought that was his fault. When she did try to have sex she had a painfully dry vagina.

She finally asked if this could be menopause, since she was having night sweats and hot flashes on and off. Her last period had been seven months before, but she had put this off to being fatigued and pushing herself ever harder in her daily workouts to try and lose weight.

On examination, her skin was a little dry, musculature and reflexes were all normal, although her Achilles tendon reflexes recovery was questionably on the slow side. There were no other signs or history of hypothyroidism. Respiratory and cardiovascular systems intact as was the neurological exam.

Her basic lab tests came back normal: no anemia, electrolytes normal. Her thyroid TSH was high normal. The testosterone, free and total, were low, as were her estrogen, progesterone, and SHBG (Sex Hormone Binding Globulin). She did have very mild osteopenia as shown by the bone mass density screening.

She was clearly in menopause. I also considered the possibility of hypothyroidism, which is quite frequent in menopausal women, because of the weight gain, slow recovery of the Achilles tendon test, and dry skin. We also talked about stress since she was a Type "A" business person and under pressure from work as well as the stress of not wanting to be menopausal. In addition, any deviation because of debilitating body changes is itself a major stress factor, as is the interruption of one's way of life and relationships.

I started her on testosterone, estradiol, and progesterone bio-identical cream, which is available at compounding pharmacies. I talked to her about hypothyroidism and balancing all the hormones, but wanted to get further thyroid tests first. We talked about the wonders of passing into a beautiful new life for women and I suggested some reading material. Christiane Northrup MD's books are wonderful. This led into a discussion of stress and many ways of alleviating it, such as yoga and counseling, which Natalie was open to doing. I suggested my favorite counseling practices—hypnosis and/or Interactive Guided Imagery, since they had been so helpful to me.

At our four week follow up she was a different woman. I ordered repeats of the sex hormone tests and discussed the results of her thyroid tests, which were fine. I recommended that we recheck them in six to twelve months, depending on her symptoms and signs. She had been reading Christiane Northrup MD and was on a new path. Her libido was up and intercourse no longer painful. She and her husband were feeling a new surge in romance together.

As is abundantly clear by now, it is necessary for all the hormones to be in balance, not only the sex hormones, but also thyroid and cortisol. Some healers like to do all replacements at one time; I prefer to do some and see if alleviating all or some of the symptoms and signs brings them into equilibrium.

There are three forms of estrogen that are natural to the body: Estrone (E1), esradiol (E2) and estriol (E3). As is shown on the diagram (Appendix II), many of these hormones can convert from one form to another. This is true even if they are in different categories, or different types of hormones. Testosterone can convert to estradiol, DHEA to testosterone or estrogen, and so on. The body usually seems to know what it needs and provides it.

Estrogen is the female hormone that eventually gives the female child the feminine characteristics. All the characteristics of this hormone, as well as the problems of excess or deficiency, are listed in Appendix I. For our purpose here we need to look at just a few of the estrogen effects.

Estrogen, like testosterone, is a bone builder. This is one of the reasons why when a woman reaches perimenopause and estrogen starts to decline, she starts to lose bone density. If the bone density gets too low (measured by bone mass density) she develops osteopenia and later on this can progress to the more serious osteoporosis.

As we have seen, the production of many hormones—including estrogen—is curtailed by the stress response. A woman may believe that she is living a healthy lifestyle—she may exercise regularly and follow a decent diet—yet may still lose bone density and wonder why. The cause may be continuous stress. If she is not following a healthy diet, her stress may encourage her to eat foods that can further damage her bones, for example, sodas and fast/processed foods that are more likely to be acidic. A lot of meat also creates acidity in the body. In an attempt to buffer this acidity, the body leaches calcium from the bones.

As many women have discovered, stress can alter the hormonal balance. This is especially noticeable around menstruation. Stress can alter the number of days between periods, make them heavier, make them shorter or do away with them altogether. Often, female athletes undergoing intense training stop menstruating. Don't forget we are not just talking about mental stress, but also physical stress and environmental stress. The driven athlete is not only subjecting herself to physical stress through intense training, but also in the drive to become trim, she may be following a low fat diet and restricting or eliminating the cholesterol that is a precursor to all the sex hormones. Also, if she is eating too much meat in order to gain muscle, she may be calling in the bone buffer system of calcium to rectify her acid-base balance.

Environmental stress is also a factor in depleting estrogen levels. There are many chemicals in the environment that attach to the same receptors to which natural estrogen should be attaching. Plastics are a great example, called phthalates for those wanting to delve further. These form "estrogen mimickers." Estrogen mimickers have been responsible for early menses and early maturation of females. There is also strong evidence of plastics being carcinogenic. We do know that estrogen mimics do not perform the same functions that nature wanted for the human estrogen.

Plastics are everywhere; our children live in a plastic world. Babies are put to sleep on plastic sheets, fed with plastic bottles and cups and nipples, given plastic pacifiers and plastic toys. It is even possible to measure the amount of plastic—and estrogen mimics—out-gassing from the plastic wraps around our vegetables and meats. Minute amounts to be sure, but like the famous dripping water of Chinese water torture they can add up over time to cause cancers and other unknown problems, as can the growth hormones fed to poultry, dairy and meats. We are assured that it's, "Just a little bit." Yes, but the long term cumulative effects of numerous different environmental toxins are not yet known, and I think it is self evident that it won't be good. Let's say that mercury has an effect in most people at a certain level, but not everyone; but what happens when you add lead, and/or a little arsenic from wood chips treated with an arsenic preservative. Add toxins from second hand smoke, and so on. The additive effect of all these environmental toxins may affect the DNA-RNA, or cause neuropathy, and so on.

The good news is that we can make lifestyle choices that can reverse past damage and maintain a healthy balance for the future: a diet that is high in fresh fruits and vegetables; whole grains; hormone and antibiotic-free meats; regular exercise; plenty of rest, choosing non-GMO products. And what else? Stress management! Taking time each day for deep relaxation. Also making the time—with a counselor if necessary—to identify sources of stress and brainstorm ways of reducing or responding differently.

I mention identifying sources of stress because so many of us believe that it is part of life and "I can handle it;" or when such and such happens I will get out of this stress situation. Sometimes tomorrow does not come, or it comes too late. Too often we either accept the stress or do not even recognize it. We have no idea why we feel sick and tired.

In addition to the stress management aids already mentioned: counseling, hypnosis, Interactive Guided Imagery, here are two techniques I have learned that help me. One is doing "Morning Pages," recommended by Julia Cameron in her book *The Artist's Way*. First thing in the morning you write whatever comes to mind. Julia recommends three pages written by hand. I find that one page typed at the computer works for me. Grammar and spelling do not matter, it's a matter of getting stuff out of your head and onto the paper or computer.

The second is to learn self-hypnosis (from a qualified hypnotherapist) so that you can sit still and relax deeply on command.

Progesterone is the first of the woman's sex hormones to decline at perimenopause, the often uncomfortable phenomenon which many western women experience. It appears not to be experienced to the same degree by women in the east, perhaps because menopause in eastern cultures does not have a negative connotation or the expectation of uncomfortable symptoms. Also, women in the east—until recently anyway—tend to follow a diet that includes more vegetables, and less meat and dairy, especially with synthetic hormones. Vegetables contain phytohormones, natural hormones from plants that may keep a better balance during life changes. And another factor may be that at one time the women of eastern cultures were not exposed to as many environmental estrogen mimickers throughout their lives.

Perimenopause is the beginning of menopause. The obvious signs and symptoms are: mood swings; hot flashes; night sweats; bloating and weight gain; loss of libido; and for some, constant depression. Why? It is this thing called "estrogen dominance."

It is important to understand this term that is often thrown around without explanation. Most people use it to mean having a lot of estrogen, which may or may not be the case. Probably not! Because when there is insufficient progesterone to counter the effects of estrogen (each hormone has a protective alter hormone that operates a check and balance system), it can take only minimal amounts of estrogen to become dominant and give the effects of too much estrogen. This is why when a woman is given estrogen whether after a hysterectomy (could be seen as traumatic menopause) or biological menopause she must be given progesterone as well in a physiological dose to balance the estrogen. Too often, unfortunately, women who have hysterectomies—which is an unnatural and premature menopause that can be even more traumatic than a natural menopause—are often not given a balance of natural hormones.

This estrogen dominance can happen in males also. With males it is seen when they no longer produce their individual physiological testosterone but are still producing their small amount of estrogen. Or when they take too much testosterone, especially synthetics, and the body converts it to estrogen. It also happens to males when the Sex Hormone Binding Globulin (SHBG) is high enough to bind up the testosterone, whether the testosterone is naturally produced, synthetic or bio-identical. The conversion of testosterone to estrogen in the male (aromatization by the aromatase enzyme) is dangerous when the liver is not functioning properly, which renders the liver inept at ridding the body of the unwanted estrogen. This can cause high estrogen levels, which is now considered the culprit of prostate cancer. The aromatase enzyme is predominantly produced by the fat cells and therefore overweight and obese males are considered at higher risk for this testosterone-to-estrogen conversion.

Excess alcohol is a liver antagonist. Under prolonged stress, many of us self-medicate with alcohol. Heavy drinking pollutes the liver; the liver keeps the body in balance, which includes ridding the body of excess estrogen. Alcohol not only damages the liver and hinders the liver's ability to rid the body of excess estrogen; estrogen also contributes to excess weight. And the problem with excess fat—for the purposes of our primary focus in this chapter—is that the fat cell, as mentioned above, is where most of the aromatase enzyme is working, converting testosterone to estrogen. It is a vicious cycle: alcohol, causing liver problems and fat gain, gone on to set the climate for more aromatase and conversion of testosterone to estrogen.

It is interesting to note that, theoretically, the aromatase enzyme and the SHBG hormone in the female was probably a positive evolutionary development, a protective mechanism that kept the female from having too much testosterone (so she did not look like we males, luckily). The aromatase enzyme converted the excess testosterone and the SHBG tied it up so it was useless. As with the male, also in the female, if her liver is functioning poorly, then the mechanism for ridding the body of excess estrogen is defaulted and the estrogen keeps circulating in greater quantities then nature wanted. This is one of the cofactors of breast and uterine cancer: too much unused and unnecessary estrogen.

Once again, where are we going when chronic stress is part of this picture? High cortisol levels, or/and constant cortisol levels increase aromatase enzymes via fat production, which then creates more estrogens. Remember that cortisol is innately diurnal, not produced in high quantities throughout the day. At the same time, cortisol will decrease progesterone, one of whose functions is to balance estrogen. Both of these events cause estrogen dominance. It has been found that giving a woman natural progesterone can inhibit the expression of aromatase (Schmidt et al 1998).

Progesterone, like all the other sex hormones, has receptor sites on more then just the female sex organs. It has been shown through experiments on both rats and humans that it is brain protective. Women who have had severe brain injury and have been taking progesterone are released from the hospital on the average of three days sooner then those not taking progesterone. It was discovered that progesterone is necessary in helping regenerate the myelin sheath around the neurons (brain nerve cells). The myelin sheath is the outer covering of the nerves that lets impulses be transmitted quickly, sort of like insulation around an electric wire. I wonder if this would be an effective treatment for multiple sclerosis, which is a disease where the myelin sheath is lost.

Most of us (including medical students) believe that the sex hormones are only in our gonads, but this is not true. Researchers are constantly finding receptors for testosterone, estrogen and progesterone in other parts of the body, including the brain and the heart. It seems the greater source of our creation did not make each of these hormones to do just one thing, as is taught to so many practitioners. There are constant new discoveries for all these hormones and what effects they have on the body. The body's delicate hormonal balance and all its ramifications are not yet completely understood, but we do know that stress can interfere with the balance. That is why, when we let stress get the best of us for long periods of time, we are compromising our health, letting dis-ease enter, and causing earlier aging than necessary.

Hormonal imbalance affects different people in different ways. Each individual has different genetics, and any dis-ease or hormonal imbalance can affect one person differently from another. That is why it is important to find a physician who can spend time with you as an individual.

CHAPTER 5

Diabetes and the Metabolic Syndrome

OSCAR IS A 47-YEAR-OLD WHITE male; he enters the office and sits down with a heavy sigh. He is obviously overweight, but his weight is not why he is here. He has been to another doctor who told him to start thinking about his weight.

The doctor also discussed with Oscar the results of his blood tests. He told Oscar that his total cholesterol was too high at 240 mg/dl; his triglycerides were 160, LDL 170, HDL 70. Therefore he prescribed Lipitor to take down his cholesterol.

"The doc said everything else is fine, including my blood sugar which is 98."

"And how are you feeling?"

"Well, my wife says that my face is often red, and I get headaches in the back of my head. I do feel tired a lot of the time, but my job is pretty demanding and I have to fly a lot. And you know how stressful flying is today!"

"Sure do. Anything else you want to tell me?"

"I have to urinate a lot, and as I told the other doc I feel thirsty a lot of the time."

"And what do you drink when you're thirsty?"

He grinned. "Well, water tastes okay so I drink it sometimes, but I prefer Coke."

"How many Cokes a day do you think you drink?"

"Oh, I guess between three and five. Yeah, I know. I want to diet but besides loving food I am hungry so much more than I used to be. And before you ask me no, I do not have time to exercise. I used to be quite athletic up to about six years ago when I finally landed this good paying job. I hardly have time for the two kids now."

"No time for the kids, huh? And what about your wife? How's your sex life?"

He shook his head. "What sex life? To be honest I'm not that interested any more, maybe because I'm so tired all the time. I don't do much more than look any more."

"And what about your social life?"

"Well, I see clients all the time and have lunch and suppers with them. Yeah, I also drink with them; it's just good business. Besides I really love rum and cokes. You know, cuba libres?"

"Do you smoke?"

He laughed. "No, doc, I don't. Finally something I have the right answer to!"

There are several aspects of Oscar's history and physical that should ring alarm bells. Even though his blood sugar level is within normal limits, it is at the very top, and could indicate that he is pre-diabetic or already diabetic. In view of his obesity it is advisable to order a fasting insulin level. If the fasting insulin level is high, it indicates that he is trying to combat high sugar by increasing insulin in an attempt to keep his blood sugar level down. Remember, it is the job of insulin to keep the blood sugar level down.

Insulin is needed to force the sugar in the blood into the cells where it is needed. If there is too much sugar for the cells' needs, the sugar will be converted into fat. This is one of the ways that nature tries to keep us in homeostasis. When sugar levels are too high, the pancreas continues to produce insulin until the cells get tired of getting hit with insulin and we have insulin resistance. When the pancreas eventually fatigues out and does not produce insulin any more we have a case of Diabetes II.

Therefore Oscar at this point, if the insulin level is high, should be treated for diabetes, even though his blood sugar is within normal limits—just. Some would call this Pre-Diabetes, but why wait for full-blown diabetes? Treatment could be a good diet and regular exercise regimen. The awareness of what happens to people with moderate to severe diabetes can be a good motivator in this situation. The other hints that he already has diabetes are his excessive thirst (polydipsia), constant hunger (polyphagia) and frequent urination (polyuria). These are the three signs of untreated diabetes.

His high blood pressure could also be treated with exercise, diet and daily relaxation. It would be advisable for him to stay on the BP medicine if the BP is moderate to severe until his improved lifestyle allows him to get off of the medicine, and hopefully by this stage he recognizes that this is the goal. Too often, patients on medication believe it is okay to continue an unhealthy way of life since advertisements falsely persuade people that pharmaceuticals are a panacea.

At the same time, the above regimen will help Oscar's cholesterol, even though his total cholesterol is not so bad since his HDLs (good cholesterol) are so good. Remember, you want the HDL, or good cholesterol, to be higher than 45, so Oscar's HDL of 70 is very, very good. The total cholesterol is the sum of the HDL's and LDL's (bad cholesterol—see chapter 3), so a high HDL like Oscar's will skew the total cholesterol upward, just like we see here with Oscar's total cholesterol of 240. His LDL's are concerning, however, at 170, which is greater than the accepted norm of 100.

And of course, Oscar needs to stop drinking Coke, since each one has the equivalent of ten teaspoons of sugar. If three to five Cokes a day does not sound like that many to you, how would you feel about eating thirty to fifty teaspoons of sugar a day?

Oscar presents the classic symptoms of Metabolic Syndrome, once known as Syndrome X, a stress-related disease that is becoming so prevalent in the western world that the number of cases is increasing at a rate higher than new cases of AIDS; about forty seven million Americans have Metabolic Syndrome; that is about one in four people.

As is clear from Oscar, excess weight is part of the Metabolic Syndrome package. He loves food, but he also eats and drinks more than he probably would otherwise because of business expectations. Under stress many people over eat. Nervous eating, eating anything and everything when we're not hungry, or craving a particular food such as chocolate or ice cream, is the way many of us seek to soothe ourselves when the emotional vampires—the pressures and demands of life—crowd in on us. When we are under time pressure we tend to eat the worst kind of foods: fast food or processed food that is relatively inexpensive and easy, but is low in nutrition and high in the worst kind of fat. And when restaurant meals are a frequent part of doing business, as is the case for Oscar, or more convenient because of time pressures, as we know they usually involve mammoth portions of everything, and often copious amounts of alcohol.

Metabolic Syndrome is also being seen in our children. At this point in time it is estimated that about one million teenagers have Metabolic Syndrome. Stressed parents tend to overfeed their children, perhaps in a misguided attempt to compensate for being stressed. We tend to offer food as a panacea or a peace offering for hurt feelings or lack of quality time. Stressed parents don't have the time to shop for and cook live food that contains vitamins, minerals, healthy fats, and complex carbohydrates. Add to this the fact that many of our children play video games a lot more than baseball or football or soccer; and spend hours per day watching TV, when they are often also snacking on empty calorie foods. One can of soda can have as much as ten teaspoons of sugar, and it is not unusual for a young person to consume two or three of these a day, just like Oscar. Interestingly, overweight parents frequently do not perceive their children as being overweight.

As mentioned, Oscar's frequent thirst, in conjunction with his other symptoms, is a red flag for diabetes, and he is trying to quench his thirst with a drink that is exacerbating his symptoms, quite apart from the high caloric content of Coke. There are warning signs of diabetes—polydipsia (excessive thirst), polyphagia (overeating), and polyuria (excessive urination). And at business meetings he is drinking rum with Coke, a double whammy. Diabetes is often related to obesity and hypertension, which make up part of the Metabolic Syndrome. While much of the world suffers from the lack of food, we in the West are killing ourselves with an abundance of the wrong type of food. This may be the first generation of children with a shorter life expectancy than their parents.

Alcohol consumption can be another factor in the development of Metabolic Syndrome. As we seek comfort and relief in our stress-saturated society many of us turn to alcohol (that has a high sugar content) as well as the sugary pacifiers mentioned above. And the negative effects of sugar in the body go beyond the obvious weight gain, or rather feed into a complicated feedback mechanism that compounds the weight gain.

Serotonin receptors in the body accept the sugar as if it were serotonin, similar to the way in which phthalates (plastics) fool the receptors for estrogen, as we saw in chapter 4. The job of serotonin is to keep us calm; this is why serotonin modifiers are prescribed for sufferers of depression and bipolar disorder. The medications are called Selective Serotonin Reuptake Inhibitors [SSRIs]; they inhibit the re-absorption of serotonin, so that serotonin levels in the blood remain higher, keeping the mood elevated. Consumption of alcohol and sugar foods provides a similar serotonin effect, because the serotonin receptors are being tied up by the sugar, leaving more serotonin in the blood, but it is short lived, and therefore more is required to counteract the down feeling.

Refined sugars enter the bloodstream very quickly and provide a "sugar high," a temporary feeling of wellbeing. The problem, though, is that the blood sugar levels drop just as precipitately, often below what is considered normal and healthy, inducing a hypoglycemic state with symptoms of feeling tired, depressed or angry. This is not true hypoglycemia but rather an induced low sugar state from the quick drop due to the sudden insulin surge. (We will explore the stress/insulin mechanism in a moment.) It is called reactive hypoglycemia.

The adrenal gland responds to this reactive hypoglycemia by putting out adrenaline and cortisol, because—once again—the body responds to the reactive hypoglycemia as it responds to any stress, as if it were a flight or fight situation. The brain is dependent on sugar to function, therefore low blood sugar equals stress. It is the adrenaline rush of the stress response that leads to the sympathetic reaction of hunger, nervousness, feeling faint, heart palpitations and even tremors. We tend to crave more sugar in order to get that serotonin savior back.

As we well know by now, prolonging the stimulus of adrenaline and cortisol eventually causes adrenal fatigue and very low production of cortisol. Stress brings on this cascade of insulin activity that is further complicated by the sympathetic response of hunger. We crave sugar, eat it, and temporarily feel better. But it is excess sugar that perpetuates the Metabolic Syndrome.

There is also evidence that low levels of the neurotransmitter dopamine are involved with depression or just feeling "low." Dopamine stimulates the reward center of the brain, and it has a relationship with insulin. Normal insulin levels seem to stimulate the release of dopamine and therefore keep us on an even keel, while high insulin or insulin resistance lower dopamine levels. When dopamine levels are low and we feel down, we eat sugary and fatty foods in order to get that dopamine feeling and feel good again (Kash & Lombard, 2008). In other words, low dopamine due to high insulin stimulates the body and brain to have food cravings, while normal insulin levels produce physiological (normal) levels of dopamine and the person feels good. Emotional vampires—the various sources of stress in our lives—stimulate the stress response that influences an increased insulin production. Please see the diagram on cortisol, blood sugar, and insulin.

Let's review the role of insulin in the stress response.

The stress response releases more cortisol from the adrenals. The cortisol tells the liver that we are under attack and need fuel to cope with the situation, to fight or to run. The liver obliges by dumping its stores of sugar (the fuel) into the blood stream. The elevated blood sugar levels tell the pancreas that more insulin is needed so that the sugar can get into the cells where it can be used.

If we are indeed fighting someone or running away, all well and good. We fight or run, and then everything goes back to normal. But when the stress is chronic, meaning it is constant or occurs in frequent bursts, the continuous outpouring of sugar from the liver causes a constant outpouring of insulin from the pancreas. The insulin receptors of the cells cannot handle all that sugar, so it is deposited as fat for future use. This is how stress can sabotage even the most committed dedication to a weight loss, diet, and exercise program. This fat is deposited in the abdominal area in men, and, in women, first in the buttocks and thighs, then eventually in the abdomen.

If insulin output continues at a high rate, eventually the cell receptors for insulin get tired of being hit and start to resist. This is the stage of insulin resistance that is pre-diabetic. The pancreas, in an effort to get the sugar into the cells where it can do some good, puts out higher and higher amounts of insulin, and the cells continue to resist, so the sugar cannot get into the cells and remains in the blood. Eventually the blood sugar levels rise to the problem we call diabetes II. The problem is not that a diabetic has too little sugar; it is that the sugar is not in the right place to be used by the body: the cells.

Insulin, like all hormones, does its job efficiently only if it is in physiological quantities. At high levels insulin is toxic to the arteries. When the body's cells do not receive the proper glucose (sugar)—because insulin resistance is keeping it locked out of the cells so that it stays in the blood—they cannot function properly. As we have seen, nature turns a lot of the excess sugar into triglycerides (fat). The arterial cells, especially the inner lining that is called the endothelium, are going through the same trauma as other cells in the body in regard to the high fats floating through the blood. The fat, especially the LDL or bad fats, seeps into the endothelium, which is the lining of the blood cells. This occurs especially in the arterial area where there is inflammation and, therefore, opening for this infiltration to occur.

This fat should not be there, in the endothelium, and is therefore considered an invasion. The body's response to invasion is to mobilize the immune system, which in this case releases an army of white blood cells known as "macrophages." The macrophages ingest the LDL, oxidize, and die. They become a toxic hazard inside the endothelium. This signals other macrophages to come and clean up the mess and the same thing happens to them. Those macrophages that have done their job and ingested the LDL's are now called "foam cells" because they are so bloated with fat. Eventually, there is such a build-up that the internal arterial circumference is compromised, narrowing the blood vessel and elevating blood pressure. Eventually this build-up compromises the integrity of the arterial wall, so that the fat seeps out, causing fatty streaks and hardening of the artery when joined by calcium, leading to still higher blood pressure and restriction of blood flow.

The stress response—to the job in Oscar's case, or to any one or combination of the myriad stresses that are a fact of modern life—especially when combined with a stress-related high sugar diet, set in motion a cascade of events that promotes hardening of the arteries (atherosclerosis). This is why people with diabetes have 3-4 times the problems of atherosclerosis than those without. This brings on hypertension and peripheral artery disease (PAD) with all of their attendant complications to the organs and tissues of the body, including heart attacks and strokes.

Metabolic Syndrome (Syndrome X)

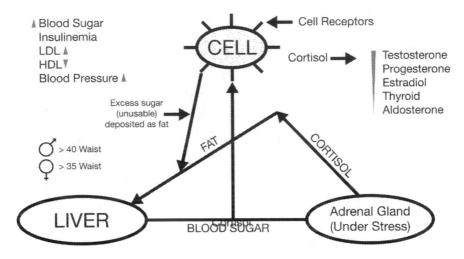

For more information on all the other functions of insulin that have been recently discovered, I highly recommend a great and easy to read book called *Freedom from Disease*, by Peter Kash and Jay Lombard, D.O.

This is how the Metabolic Syndrome develops, as a result of a high stress life and a diet high in sugar and unhealthy fat and low in nutrition, lack of exercise, lack of down time and so on. The signs and symptoms of Metabolic Syndrome are:

- hyperlipidemia (too many fats in the body)
- high blood pressure
- hyperinsulinemia (high insulin levels)
- high triglycerides and LDL cholesterol (bad cholesterol)
- low HDL cholesterol (good cholesterol)
- a waist measurement in a man of more than 40 inches and a woman more than 35 inches.

There are variations of this syndrome, of course, but these are the classic signs and symptoms. So what can be done about it? The remedy is in following the prescription for a healthy lifestyle in chapter 8: learning how to respond in a healthier way to stressful situations; regular exercise; a healthy diet; and daily relaxation. But, like Oscar, many patients are resistant to the idea of making lifestyle changes and all too often sufferers of Metabolic Syndrome are treated with statin drugs (such as Lipitor, Mevacor, Zocor) and antidepressants (SSRIs such as Lexapro, Effexor, Paxil, Prozac, Zoloft) with all their side effects. In my opinion this is like applying a Band-Aid to a major laceration.

Stress creates or contributes to the development of dis-ease, and if the causes are not remedied the dis-ease itself compounds the stress and exacerbates the problem, in a kind of toxic feedback mechanism. There are emotional, social and physical stresses when one has diabetes and/or the Metabolic Syndrome, such as the embarrassment or social censure experienced by those who are overweight. We see the debate about overweight people on airlines going on right now. There is also the potential for more stress from the side effects of medications. The cholesterol lowering statin drugs, as we saw in Chapter 3, can cause liver problems and deplete the body of CoQ10, necessary for the cells to make energy, especially the heart. They can also cause muscle breakdown (Rhabdomyolysis) that can be permanent if the drug is not stopped immediately, and now they have been implicated in dementia. The SSRI drugs (for depression) can cause tiredness, worsening depression in some cases, sexual dysfunction, weight gain and insomnia. These are just a few of the side effects. Don't you think all of these would make one more depressed and stressed?

I am not presenting the medicinal solutions, whether they are allopathic or alternative, since this book is not about medicines or botanicals, but rather how and why we get into the hormonal imbalance. However, I do think it is important to know that many natural remedies do exist. I have used botanicals along with lifestyle change for clients for many years with successful results. But I know, from my own health challenges and those of my patients, that if one wishes to get to the cause of dis-ease stress management is mandatory. Yoga, meditation, sports and exercise can give relief and relaxation, but ultimately the cause needs to be uncovered and dealt with. The best way I can recommend is to find a non-judgmental, unconditionally loving counselor. I would recommend someone who also practices hypnosis and/or interactive guided imagery. You can check the website of the Academy for Guided Imagery for a qualified practitioner near you: www.AcademyforGuidedImagery.com

Hypnosis and imagery are tools that allow access to the deeper levels of the mind, and can not only get to the core of the problem relatively quickly, but also recruit the vast resources of the deeper levels of the mind to offer solutions.

There is a place and need for pharmaceuticals, but I believe they should usually be a last resort, or used as a temporary remedy to give relief while the necessary adjustments to lifestyle are made and while seeking understanding and healthier solutions to the sources of stress in our lives. Whichever road you choose to travel, I believe that with Metabolic Syndrome—as with all the imbalances we are discussing—the most beneficial path is to get to the reason why this is happening and learn how to change the circumstances. Metabolic Syndrome is a set-up for many potentially serious illnesses: arteriosclerosis, cardiovascular disease, stroke, and diabetes with all of its co-morbidities, and yes, even Alzheimer's Disease. People with Metabolic Syndrome have a seventy percent greater chance of developing Alzheimer' Disease than those without it.

What I am stressing here (no pun intended) is that there are many things one can do to improve physical health and quality of life; but one must include ways of alleviating the everyday vampires of stress along with diet, exercise and the silver bullet of learning to relax. Easier said then done. I am still working on this last point and find it invigorating when I neutralize another emotional vampire. I needed help; luckily for me my wife is in the field of stress management. What? Did you think I just know all this stuff?

When I see a "high normal" sugar level it signals that the person may be in a state of prediabetes and I order a fasting blood sugar along with a fasting insulin level. If the insulin level is high it signifies that the body is trying to compensate by keeping the sugar down and masking that the sugar would be higher if not for this compensation. I prefer to treat the person as if they have diabetes at this point in order to avoid the development of true, full-blown Type II Diabetes.

CHAPTER 6

Weight Management and Stress

As mentioned in the previous chapter, we often turn to the pacification of food when stressed. Food is the fuel that powers the body; it gives us energy for healing, for growth, for thought, for movement, and for emotional expression. Ideally we would consume only as much as the body requires to fulfill those needs.

However, as a culture, we have developed complicated rituals and beliefs around food, many of which have nothing to do with our bodies' fuel requirements. We eat for enjoyment, for social interaction, at business meetings, for comfort, for the sensual sensations associated with the tastes and textures of food, for many reasons that have nothing to do with satisfying hunger.

Many of us as children were offered a cookie or ice cream when we fell and scraped our knees and the belief that food is comfort has pursued us into our adult lives so that when we are stressed, anxious, or depressed we turn to the pacification of food.

For all of these reasons, and probably many others, many of us eat more than we need. At the same time we do not exercise enough, often because of perceived lack of time, another common vampire. This combination has resulted in an epidemic of excess weight in our culture. We spend vast amounts of money on weight-loss programs and diet pills that promise we can continue to eat whatever we want and still lose weight, but many of us have learned that fad diets don't work in the long term. They may help us lose weight temporarily, but most people gain back what they have lost, and even more, as soon as they come off the diet.

One of the problems already mentioned are the types of foods we eat when depressed, which are usually foods that are bad for our health. It is almost like epicurean suicide. These foods are marketed as comfort foods because the sugar and fat content make you feel temporarily mentally satisfied due to the serotonin effect described in Chapter 5. However, many of us pay for the temporary feeling of wellbeing induced by higher levels of serotonin with the cravings that follow when the blood sugar level drops and—very often—the additional stress of guilt. "Why did I do that?" we say to ourselves, as we look at the cheese cake crumbs or the empty package of potato chips. We feel guilty about "pigging out" and therefore depressed, so we rationalize that we may as well hang for a sheep as a lamb and eat more snacks or unhealthy food.

It is not just eating empty calories that cause health problems. If one is eating a lot of dead food all day there is not room for live food, which exacerbates the health problems and leads to more stress. It becomes a vicious cycle. Many of these cycles can be broken when we figure out what is causing the "me" who doesn't feel like me to do these disruptive things. This is why I keep emphasizing stress management as a good diving board to jump off; a competent stress management counselor will help you to uncover the unconscious motivations for self-destructive behaviors.

"Dead" foods are foods that do more harm then good: simple carbohydrates—white bread, white sugar, white rice; fried foods, processed foods, trans fat foods, and sugar under all the different names it is called under the required contents: fructose, corn syrup, sucrose, are among the many and varied names for sugar. I believe most things in plastic snack bags and most white food are probably not healthy.

I would not give too much credence to the FDA food pyramid since some fats are healthy and some are not and the FDA pyramid does not distinguish between the two. Unfortunately, all too often the government is looking after big business, such as dairy and beef, and not your health. Even the FDA's Recommended Daily Allowance (RDA) on vitamin pills is way off the path of what a good vitamin intake should be. At a medical lecture once I heard RDA defined as "Really Dumb Advice." If a vitamin is in one or two capsules per day there are probably not enough vitamins in it; usually it will take three to four capsules twice a day to acquire a sufficient amount. Remember, vitamins and most supplements are just that—supplements. Good nutrition is the key to health; a supplement cannot compensate for poor dietary intake.

"Live" food is easy. They are the foods on which mankind always survived until the advent of processed foods and advertising about seventy years ago. Organic, of course, is always the best since it eliminates insecticides, fungicides, pesticides, hormones, and antibiotics, which are all chemicals that stress the body. A variety of colors on your plate, organic or not, will mean a variety of fruits and vegetables that are beneficial for the body.

Although we have canine teeth and incisors, primitive man probably never ate a lot of meat, since primitive hunting tools were not very efficient. In primitive hunter-gatherer societies meat from the hunt was cause for a protein party, but the staples of day to day survival were the foods that were gathered, probably by the women: berries, edible plants and roots. When the hunters did succeed in bringing an animal home to the tribe, everybody probably gorged themselves since they did not know when the opportunity would arise again. Therefore, like other animals, we have evolved a gene that drives us to eat in bounty when it is available.

The problem is that, in general, there is no longer any need for this gene in our western society but it still stimulates this gorging behavior in many of us. This is why buffets are dangerous. Another factor to consider is that animals in Paleolithic times did not carry much fat. Some estimate that at that time animals carried about 4% body fat as compared to the 30% fat content of today's commercially raised beef (Boyd & Konneg, 1985).

I am not against eating meat. I believe that almost anything in moderation is okay for most people, but with meat and milk I am a strong advocate of organic products. The antibiotics and growth hormones fed to commercially raised animals become concentrated in the animal's tissues and then in the tissues of those who eat them, which stresses the body. In fact, many countries around the world will not import meat from the US because of all the hormones and antibiotics fed to the animals.

It is recommended that meat protein not be more than one third of the food on your plate, and about the size of a pack of cards. The other two thirds should be complex carbohydrates—fruits and vegetables in a variety of colors. Compare that with the tendency in our culture to eat vast quantities of meat, and perhaps French Fries or a baked potato, white bread, and salad mostly composed of iceberg lettuce that has near zero nutrition, often slathered in Ranch dressing that is high in calories and saturated fat. It has been found, incidentally, that diets high in saturated fats (animal fats) promote the consumption of eating more even when a person is sated.

There is another danger in a diet high in meat protein. We now know that it is inflammation of the arterial walls that is the vampire for heart disease and not just cholesterol. One of the biggest causes of inflammation is the oxidation, or decay of LDL (the bad cholesterol). The LDL is worsened by saturated fat from red meat and dairy products.

Another reason why red meat should be eaten only in moderation, if one chooses to eat meat, is that red meat promotes the formation of homocysteine. There are many publications about homocysteine acting as a corrosive force on the endothelial lining of the arteries (the inside lining of the arteries that lets blood flow smoothly). All these cofactors that may seem complicated are promoters that cause the immune system to overreact and cause inflammation. The overreaction of our immune system is a factor in cardiovascular damage.

Meat also causes the blood to be acidic. To counteract the acidity the blood draws calcium and phosphorous from the bones to buffer the acid. This is another cofactor for the problem of osteopenia and osteoporosis in some people, especially women. Remember that there are other cofactors aside from diet, as I've previously mentioned, in the development of osteoporosis such as stress and the resultant increase in cortisol production, and steroid medications like prednisone. Refer back to Chapter 4 if you need to review.

And the overweight plot thickens. Adipose tissue, another term for fat tissue, produces hormones such as aromatase that changes testosterone to estrogen, and an inflammatory substance called tumor necrosis factor, and estrogen, all of which can be harmful to the body when produced in higher quantities than a normal physiological dose. The more adipose tissue, the greater the production of these three hormones.

Adipose tissue also produces a substance called leptin. The function of leptin is to tell the hypothalamus, which is in the brain, to signal the stomach when it is time to stop eating. The messenger that carries out this function is a substance produced by the hypothalamus called AMP-activated protein kinase (AMPK). AMPK, triggered by leptin, signals the body to stop eating and start to burn fat and glucose. This leaves room for more glucose and fat to be stored when excess occurs, which helps to prevent insulin resistance (see Chapter 5). When a person is overweight and puts out constant leptin, they will eventually get leptin resistance, which is similar to insulin resistance. The constant, elevated levels of leptin cause burn out of the leptin receptors, meaning that the leptin can no longer be used by the body to turn off the signal and stop eating.

There is another protein-chemical reaction that happens from consumption of animal products (meat and dairy) known as PTP1B. Elevated levels of PTP1B, from eating a diet high in animal products, block leptin, again halting the process of feeling sated. I must add that it was also found that monounsaturated and polyunsaturated fats (good fats, from vegetable sources) counteract the PTP1B effect by restoring leptin sensitivity. Resveratrol, found in red wine, also sensitizes the cells to leptin, which is one of the reasons why a glass of red wine can be beneficial, but this is not an excuse to drink a lot of red wine that can have other deleterious effects. Moderation in all things, I say, and so did Aristotle. This may be one of the reasons for the French paradox. The French diet is high in rich, fatty foods, but the incidence of cardiovascular problems and excess weight is not high (Schrauwan, & Westerstep, 2000).

All this scientific data may be tedious and is presented only so that the reader has a frame of reference. There is no need to memorize it all and there is no test at the end! But it highlights all the work being done to find solutions to excess weight, obesity, Metabolic Syndrome and diabetes. What is important for the purposes of this book is the degree to which excess weight stresses the body, so I will continue with the latest scientific findings.

We will start with Adiponectin, a hormone that can only be created in lean fat cells. When a person is overweight and their fat cells, which are called adipocytes, are enlarged with fat they cannot produce sufficient adiponectin. What is the importance of this hormone? A lot! The function of this big player is to stop inflammation. It stops the production of inflammatory chemicals, such as cytokines like TNF and interleukin 6, and also downgrades the production of macrophages, a type of white blood cell that we have met before in Chapter 5. Macrophages come out when there is inflammation in order to protect us, but in the long run cause buildup of plaque, which causes inflammation. Adiponectin also makes the cells more sensitive to insulin and therefore fights insulin resistance and diabetes. It can also restore insulin sensitivity, once the excess weight is lost.

Another function of adiponectin is causing cell death to abnormal cells, like cancer cells. Scientists have found that adiponectin hinders the adhesion of platelets, similar to the effects of aspirin and diminishing adhesion of platelets prevents clotting of the arteries. In fact, by counteracting inflammation, adiponectin is counteracting all the diseases connected to inflammation, such as cardiovascular disease, heart attacks, arteriosclerosis, strokes, and many other pathologic conditions.

Overeating, or eating the wrong kinds of food, is only one of the negative coping patterns with which we attempt to deal with the vampires in our lives. Some of us watch too much television, or go on spending sprees (it has a new name now: retail therapy), or release pent-up energy in emotional outbursts. And some of us turn to dependence on chemicals: drugs, both legal and illegal; cigarettes; and alcohol. We mentioned alcohol in relation to its deleterious effect on the liver, contributing to estrogen dominance in Chapter 4, and in relation to its high sugar content contributing to Metabolic Syndrome in Chapter 5. Here we are concerned with the high caloric content of alcohol contributing to excess weight.

Self-medicating with alcohol as a solution to stress is so prevalent in our culture that there is widespread reluctance to acknowledge the damage it does, to individuals and to society at large. Not infrequently a patient would tell me that they did not want to become dependent on medications, yet on further history I would discover that they were dependent on alcohol. Even though they drank a lot, they would deny being an alcoholic or dependent on alcohol since they were still able to function on the job.

I also encountered some reformed alcoholics, members of AA, who were still carrying the same problems that drove them to drink, for which they substituted antidepressants and other medications for the alcohol. This may be more socially acceptable, but does not address the underlying cause of their chemical dependency. They are still stressed and may be stressing others, and dependent on drugs to elevate their mood, control their blood pressure and other stress-related diseases we have discussed.

The concept of the "dry alcoholic" is one that is relatively new to me; in fact it was one of these emotional vampires that gave me the idea of writing this book. A dry alcoholic is someone who has given up drinking and no longer attends AA meetings, but still has the same characteristics as imbibing alcoholics. If you live with or are friends with a dry alcoholic, you will know that they are often emotional vampires dependent on making others feel guilty and using others for their own emotional gains. They still have the problems that drove them to alcohol, and may seek to control others in order to make themselves feel more powerful, in control, and righteous. They may believe in their superiority to others and believe it is their right to subjugate them, all to deflect attention away from their own emotional problems and the need to seek help in resolving them.

Alcohol-related behaviors, whether they are the consequences to the liver, to estrogen levels, or to excess weight are sources of stress for the alcoholic; the alcoholic's behaviors—both the active alcoholic and the dry alcoholic—are vampires for those around them.

As we saw in Chapter 5, simple carbohydrates that enter the blood stream quickly cause a temporary "sugar high" and feelings of wellbeing soon followed by a "sugar low" and feeling down and craving more simple carbs. There is a classification of foods and how fast they enter the blood called the glycemic index. Consumption of high glycemic foods over-stimulates the pancreatic production of insulin, causing blood sugar to fluctuate between being too high (hyperglycemia) and too low (reactive hypoglycemia). Apart from the stress response mechanism discussed in Chapter 5 leading to insulin resistance, diabetes Type II and the Metabolic Syndrome, sugar cravings lead to high consumption of high caloric foods and contribute to excess weight.

In our discussion of Metabolic Syndrome we learned about cortisol, insulin, and the conversion of excess sugar into fat. This consequence of the stress response can sabotage our efforts to lose weight, even if we are exercising and being diligent about portion size and food combinations. So, yet again, stress management is the key to weight management and general health.

As we said in the beginning, weight management is a matter of balancing intake of energy (food) with expenditure of energy. We expend energy just to stay alive, to grow and to heal, to think, to express emotion, and to move. The way to increase expenditure of energy, when we've taken in too much food, is to increase movement: yes, I'm talking about exercise. I know that's a dreaded word for a lot of people, but I hope to encourage a different attitude toward exercise: not a chore, but nurturing of self, a way of taking care of yourself, treating yourself well. In time it can come to feel like an indulgence! It is a good idea to call it "funout" instead of workout.

Unfortunately I used to hear the same thing over and over again in my practice: "I do not have time to exercise." When we consider all the benefits of exercising, and the negative consequences of not exercising, the more pertinent question might be: Can you afford not to? The bottom line is a matter of physics: you cannot lose weight, or maintain a healthy weight, if you do not burn off as many calories as you are consuming. Diet medications and fad diets that promise you anything different are, well, lying. No one, no doctor or diet guru, can wave a magic wand and change the laws of physics for you.

It can help to approach this from another direction. When someone says, "I don't have time to exercise," I ask them to think about where all their time is going: to the kids, to the spouse, to the job, to the myriad tasks that our complicated lives involve. Then I would tell them that by saying, "I do not have time for exercise," they are sending a subconscious message to their brain that they are not worth a minimum of thirty minutes a day. They are saying: The kids are worth it, my spouse is worth it, my boss is worth it, and all the big and small stress factors in my life are worth it, but I am not. I am not worth even half an hour a day to take care of me.

Think about it. Are you worth twenty to sixty minutes per day? If you honestly answer "no," then I strongly recommend that you at least make an hour a week to see a counselor about ways to improve your sense of self worth. The truth is that you are worth it. If you don't believe that, there may be judgments and criticisms from the past replaying in the depths of your subconscious that tell you, you are "supposed" to put other people first, that self sacrifice is what God wants you to do, that if you take time for yourself you are selfish and bad, and a hundred other variations on the same theme.

Once you decide that you are worth the time it takes for self nurture, then the how and when are infinitely easier to manage. Self nurture is what exercise and healthy eating are—not just one more chore to fit into a busy day, but a reward to yourself, a way of showing yourself the kindness and respect that you probably give so freely to others, a way of taking care of the precious life with which you have been gifted. It may mean getting up earlier, and if sacrificing a half hour of sleep feels like too high a price to pay, at least do yourself the favor of giving it a try. When you do, you will find that spending that half hour in meditation or exercise or a combination will give you so much more energy than an extra half hour of sleep. Or it may mean joining a spa or gym away from the house and telephone. Yes, it does take discipline at first but after a while it becomes part of your enjoyable life.

A caveat here—if you happen to be a competitive Type A personality (like me) beware of getting into some workout that becomes competitive and creates another stressful situation. I know whereof I speak. I always wanted to learn archery, and after my illness I finally had enough time to do it. I discovered an archery range and bought a recurve bow, and spent a couple of hours three times a week at the range. While I was there I was totally, uncomplicatedly happy.

I got pretty good at archery, so much so that my new friends at the range talked me into entering a competition. I entered and I started serious training to prepare for it. If I had a bad shooting day I'd come home angry and disappointed in myself; if it rained and I couldn't shoot I'd be mopey and irritable; if the archery supply company sent me the wrong size arrows I'd pitch a fit. All this happened until my wife said one day: "You know, going to the range used to make you so happy. You'd come back home glowing. You shot for the joy of it. That damn competition has ruined everything."

She was right. I withdrew from the competition and went back to shooting for fun. It was not only relaxing and enjoyable again, but I shot much better because I was more relaxed and focused. I have also discovered that if I keep a small smile on my face while working out (I'd rather call it playing out) instead of a tight "got to do it face," it makes my mind not feel competitive but rather relaxed.

Exercise does not have to be strenuous to be beneficial. It can be walking, which can also be used as a walking meditation. It can be yoga of different sorts; there are so many choices today. Some take up martial arts or T'ai Chi. If you get bored easily and wish to do cardio workouts you can mix several different activities: biking, walking, cross training machine, and so on. You can do a short period of each instead of just one or alternate days among the different types.

Another biological benefit to exercise, relevant to weight management, is that the greater the muscle mass, the more calories that are burned all the time, not only when exercising. Muscle is active tissue; it burns calories just to stay alive, whereas fat tissue just sits there. So as you build more muscle you will burn more calories to maintain the muscle tissue, even while sleeping. Building muscle, especially through weight training, increases the body's metabolic rate, so we continue to burn fat 24 hours a day; four and a half pounds of muscle burns as many calories as running a mile every day.

The recommended thirty minutes per day of exercise does not have to be continuous. Some studies have shown it can be just as beneficial when divided into three ten-minute periods throughout the day. Personally, I prefer to do it all together since I believe the endurance and cardiovascular benefits develop more in this type of workout. But whatever is convenient and enjoyable is what is best for you, and anything you do is better than a procrastination workout.

There is another bonus to exercise, besides weight management, a healthier cardiovascular system and respiratory system, toned muscles and stronger bones. Any other benefits you can think of? There are a multitude of evidence-based studies showing that exercise for 30-45 minutes per day is as effective as taking antidepressants for mild to moderate depression, and with only beneficial side effects, unlike most antidepressants. I believe this is true not only because it stimulates the body to produce endorphins (the natural chemical morphine that makes you feel good), but also because exercising often involves socializing with other people outside of the usual everyday stressful environment. People begin to feel better about doing something for themselves and simultaneously something scientifically proven to be beneficial for their health. Also their mind is taken off of the worrisome day's schedule for a while.

Perhaps most important of all, for our purposes here, exercise is a great stress reliever. The Stress Response prepares us for physical action: to fight or flee and anything involving physical exertion is going to give the body the message to return to normal. All of the negative consequences to the various vampires in our lives are mitigated through exercise. It is the single most important gift that you can give to yourself.

There are no coincidences! As I am sitting here writing this chapter, a Cancer Institute called to see if I could help them with a survey and write about the relationship between being overweight or obese and cancer, such as cancers of the breast, colon, endometrium, esophagus, kidney and prostate. "After smoking, obesity is the highest preventable cancer risk," according to the American Institute of Cancer Research and Health magazine.

I hope this does not come off as an admonishment to those who are overweight; my purpose is to examine what stress does to our society and to us. Stress is but one piece in the puzzle when it comes to overweight and there are other causes to be aware of including genetics, low thyroid hormone, and aging. What can cause low thyroid? S-t-r-e-s-s. (I know I sound like a broken record.) We will examine the thyroid in greater detail in the following chapter.

CHAPTER 7

Stress and the Thyroid

ELLEN IS 50-YEAR-OLD WOMAN WHO went to her doctor because she was feeling tired, depressed, and gaining weight. She felt cold all the time, was losing her hair and eyebrows, and was constipated. All her lab results were interpreted as within normal limits, including her thyroid stimulating hormone (TSH). Her doctor diagnosed hormonal imbalance and prescribed synthetic hormones.

This used to be the standard treatment for women her age, though hopefully not as common since the Women's Health Initiative Study showed deleterious effects from synthetic hormones. See Chapter 4 for more information on the WHIS. The synthetic hormones did not help Ellen and a month later she returned to her doctor with the same complaints: dry skin, constipation, lethargy, hair loss, loss of the outer third of her eyebrows and a temperature below 97.4. And she was not losing weight even though she was exercising every day.

These are all the textbook signs and symptoms of hypothyroidism, but Ellen's blood work showed her thyroid-stimulating hormone (TSH) within the normal limits of .25-5.5 mU/L (milliunits per microliter—the measurement in which thyroid results are expressed.) So Ellen's doctor prescribed an antidepressant. The side effects of the antidepressant made her more tired, lowered her sex drive and made her gain more weight. Her depression felt about the same, but now she was also experiencing anxiety because of the side effects of the medication and no improvement in her symptoms. Her doctor recommended that she see a psychiatrist.

Doctors have been debating for years whether to lower the upper limit of what is considered normal for TSH (thyroid stimulating hormone) since so many people whose blood work shows their TSH close to this upper limit still have the symptoms and signs of a low thyroid. But when a busy physician takes a history of all the above symptoms and signs s/he may only hear depressed, tired and menopause and see lab results in the normal range. It would be in the patient's best interest, I believe, to consider the signs and symptoms first and the blood work second. In Ellen's case that would have been the clue that it was likely to be a thyroid problem, and a full thyroid panel could have been ordered.

As we have seen, production of many hormones, including thyroid, is lowered when the body is stressed; the Stress Response triggers the adrenal gland to produce higher levels of cortisol, that signals the body to put all its energy into the systems that will help to fight or run, and take energy away from functions that are not essential to those life-saving activities. In the case of chronic stress, the low production of thyroid hormone over time can lead to hypothyroidism.

The thyroid hormone is one of the main hormones that stimulate the furnace of the cells to produce energy. Without it, or when the thyroid hormone is low, food cannot be efficiently metabolized, so energy levels are low, and the food that cannot be used is stored as fat, which is what lead to Ellen's symptoms of fatigue and weight gain. Her signs and symptoms indicated a low thyroid and/or low cortisol, even though her lab results were within the normal range.

A low thyroid level is called hypothyroid or hypothyroidism. Hypothyroidism may also be caused by a poorly functioning adrenal gland, since too much or too little cortisol affects the thyroid gland. As we know, the adrenal gland produces cortisol and adrenaline in response to stress, and powers the Stress Response, which prepares the body to fight or flee. In the initial stages stress causes higher than normal levels of cortisol, but when the stress is chronic the adrenals eventually wear down, a condition known as "adrenal fatigue," and cortisol production drops below normal levels. Therefore there is not enough cortisol available to make the usable type of thyroid hormone.

The machinery of the body functions on precise amounts of each chemical, some measured in billionths of a milligram, and this includes the hormones. This precise amount is known as the physiological quantity. All the hormones have to be available in the appropriate physiological quantity in order to function in harmony for optimum well-being, sort of like a symphony with each musician playing exactly the right notes in harmony with all the others.

Many women entering menopause not only experience the effects of diminishing sex hormones but also have a thyroid problem, and as we saw with Ellen one of the symptoms of low thyroid hormone is depression. I believe the depression comes also from the physical changes—constipation, hair loss, feeling cold, gaining weight, fatigue—that disrupt one's life. I believe that the thyroid should always be explored before starting anyone on antidepressants. This scenario will become clearer as we continue to explore associations between the thyroid and stress. As previously mentioned, menopause can affect the thyroid—not just the sex hormones of estrogen, progesterone, and testosterone. In a case such as Ellen's, I also order tests to evaluate the sex hormones and the thyroid.

The thyroid is essential for the metabolism of our nutrient intake, and therefore the energy source for all our functions. It is stimulated by a complex hormonal feedback system to the hypothalamus and the thyroid gland via the circulation of thyroid hormone T4 (thyroxin).

The pituitary gland produces the thyroid stimulating hormone (TSH), which in turn stimulates the thyroid to produce T4. However, T4 is inactive, and must convert to active T3 in order to do its job.

The conversion from inactive T4 to active T3 requires the right amount of selenium and cortisol. If selenium and cortisol are lacking or levels are inadequate, the feedback to the pituitary gland can make the level of TSH appear normal, since the T4 is sending the message that all is okay. The physician reading the lab report sees that the TSH is within normal limits, even though the patient is deficient in T3. The deficiency of selenium may be due to a poor diet, an excess of cortisol due to early stages of chronic stress, or a deficiency in cortisol due to adrenal fatigue; in any case, not the physiological quantity of cortisol.

And the plot thickens. Under stress, T4 can convert into what is known as reverse T3 (rT3). The rT3 molecule is just like T3 (see Appendix II), except that one of the three iodine ions is in the wrong position. This tricks the receptor sites of the cells; rT3 binds to the receptors, thus blocking any remaining T3; but since the rT3 does not have the same active stimulus as T3 because it is not of the right molecular arrangement, it will not stimulate the thyroid's metabolic functions in the cells. Therefore, prescribing T4 will not solve the problem. The more synthetic T4 a patient takes the more rT3 is produced, and the patient's condition either does not improve or gets worse (Wilson, 1992).

Or let's say the patient is being treated with synthetic or natural T3 but still does not feel well. It is possible that the T3 is not getting into the cell, because to get into the cell the T3 is dependent on selenium and a physiological level of cortisol, and these may be deficient. Or if the T3 does get into the cell it may not work if zinc levels are low, because here it is dependent on zinc for its performance on the mitochondria in the cell (the multitude of little factories in the cells that produce energy).

When the stress levels rise, the enzyme which is responsible for the conversion of T4 to T3 is also used for conversion of T4 to rT3. Therefore, there is not enough of the enzyme to convert to both and rT3 seems to take precedence, for reasons that are not known at this time. The good news is that rT3 can be measured, and if it is high then supplements of natural T3 can be taken so that the conversion is not necessary.

The reason for the existence of rT3 is stress, so it is advisable to check cortisol levels—because cortisol is the stress hormone that powers the stress response—before prescribing a supplemental thyroid hormone. Or, if the patient is already taking thyroid medicine but is not getting good results, cortisol levels should be checked to determine if the patient needs cortisol supplementation along with other natural supplements, or have adrenal treatment added to the regimen. Of course stress management counseling is also advisable so that the adrenal problem will not continue.

To summarize: it is possible for a physician to be fooled by lab work. In this case, T4 levels remain normal but are not being converted to the usable T3. The feedback of the T4 from the thyroid is still telling the pituitary that all is okay and therefore the TSH (thyroid stimulating hormone) remains normal. But if the patient has all the symptoms and signs of hypothyroidism, I would say the heck with the lab work being in the normal limits. An rT3 test is needed here and maybe some other thyroid tests: T3, FT3, T4, FT4 and an autoimmune profile for thyroid.

Thyroid

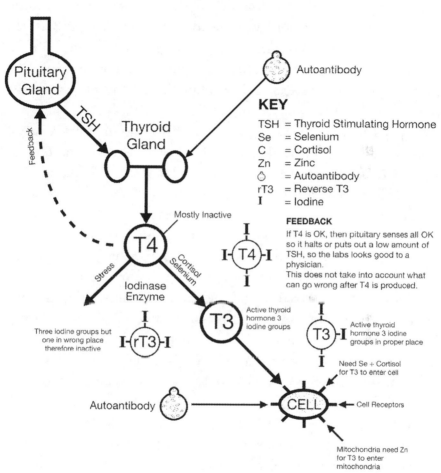

KEY

TSH = Thyroid Stimulating Hormone
Se = Selenium
C = Cortisol
Zn = Zinc
⚬ = Autoantibody
rT3 = Reverse T3
I = Iodine

FEEDBACK

If T4 is OK, then pituitary senses all OK so it halts or puts out a low amount of TSH, so the labs looks good to a physician.
This does not take into account what can go wrong after T4 is produced.

Another enigma is that high cortisol levels, as a result of stress in the initial stages, before the stage of adrenal fatigue, can lower TSH production from the pituitary, keeping it in the normal range window. If a health practitioner believes only the test results and does not hear the complaints of the patient, the treatment may be off the mark. Even if a patient has a TSH level that is considered high, low or normal according to lab standards they can still have hypothyroidism if the signs and symptoms are present.

Eventually the adrenals run down due to chronic stress and cortisol levels drop. Cortisol prepares the cell receptors to accept the T3, so once again the T3 could be there but the receptors cannot accept it because cortisol levels are too low, and the numbers can mislead a health practitioner. I tend to agree with James Wilson (*Adrenal Fatigue*) that too often it is the lab report and not the person sitting in the examining room that is the patient in the practitioner's eyes.

I put Ellen on a very low dose of natural thyroid just to see if this would help and not hurt her. I knew this was some type of hypothyroidism from her symptoms and signs, but I like to start slowly. Even though this dose of thyroid was low, it did contain a greater quantity of T3. I also ordered the tests above after two weeks, with the exception of the autoimmune test. I do the autoimmune test as a last resort, and this has paid off for the patient both financially and medically since a few times it was an autoimmune problem. After the two-week trial period she admitted happily that she was already feeling better and her depression lifted. The tests all came back as I predicted. I increased her natural thyroid medication dose a little and this time waited a month to see her again. We kept in touch during this time via telephone. She was exuberant about the improvement in her symptoms and signs and her family and work life were so much better. At this point, we started working on stress and menopause. I was a happy physician with a happy client. When I had ordered the thyroid test I had also ordered the tests on her Testosterone, estradiol, SHBG. I started her on human bioidentical hormones (including testosterone) after I was satisfied with the thyroid correction. Sometimes I do all together, but this time I did only the thyroid first due to her history. Once her hormones were balanced and in symphony, she was a happy young woman again.

After following thyroid treatment for a few months it is possible that the person is still not doing well and is continuing to show signs and symptoms of hypothyroidism. Then we must look for an autoimmune disease. An autoimmune disease is where the body attacks specific parts of itself, in this case the receptors of the cells for the T3 or the thyroid hormone itself and there are blood tests to look for this specific issue. A very common autoimmune disease is Hashimoto's disease, which seems to be genetically related, that affects the thyroid. Actually both hyper—and hypothyroidism, in many cases, may have a genetic predisposition, but a predisposition does not mean the dis-ease has to manifest. Stress management counseling can often alleviate or get rid of the signs and symptoms of a genetic disorder when coupled with proper treatments such as supplements and medications as we've mentioned above.

Other options to treatment often are non conventional medicine; sometimes alternative or complementary treatment is the way to go or in conjunction with the accepted medical treatment. Sometimes it is a simple matter of changing the diet. For example, if one is using salt with chlorine in it, or toothpaste with fluoride, this could be interfering with the iodine of the thyroid hormone. Fluoride and chloride are neighbors to iodine in the molecular charts. They can push the iodine out of the thyroid hormone. Without iodine, T4 cannot be formed. So the solution is simply to switch to iodinated sea salt or iodinated Celtic salt and stop using fluorinated toothpaste.

It has also been found that sunscreen containing MBC (4-Methylbenzylidene camphor) and BP2 (benzophenone) disrupt thyroid production in rats. The rats had high TSH and low T4, probably due to interference with the iodine part of forming T4.

Another interesting theory is that when cortisol is low the gut does not absorb normally, which can lead to leaky gut syndrome, meaning that certain large protein particles that are foreign to the body are absorbed, while other nutrients that the body requires, such as amino acids, are not absorbed. For instance, leaky gut syndrome may mean that tyrosine, an amino acid, cannot be made by the body for lack of other amino acids to make it. Tyrosine plus iodine are needed to make the thyroid hormone.

Low cortisol levels hinder the production of stomach acid; protein in the stomach is not broken down sufficiently, and amino acids that come from protein will not be produced. This leads to weaker muscles, fatigue and fewer chemical processes that depend on amino acids. These include hormone production, therefore hormones—including thyroid—will be deficient.

It is stress that eventually causes low cortisol (as a result of adrenal fatigue) which may lead to low thyroid, and a further reason why cortisol levels should be tested before initiating thyroid hormone treatment, or if the person does not respond well to treatment.

Another mechanism by which stress contributes to leaky gut syndrome is the high-sugar comfort foods that many of us indulge in when stressed. These foods can contribute to irritable bowel syndrome and/or leaky gut syndrome. In this case it could be appropriate to initiate adrenal support before thyroid medication is used, as well as supplementation to correct the intestinal problem. This is especially true for someone with Chronic Fatigue Immune Disease Syndrome (CFIDS), which may be complicated by the use of narcotics for pain. Narcotics can interfere with the production of the Adrenal Cortical Tropic Hormone (ACTH), which will negatively affect the thyroid.

Another factor in leaky gut syndrome is the following: If the gut is allowing proteins to traverse it that should not, and these proteins—that are usually blocked—are getting into the blood, allergies and autoimmune problems may arise. One of these autoimmune problems could attack the thyroid (for example Hashimoto's disease). This is an easy blood test to do when it is suspected, and it should be suspected when the patient is not responding to thyroid treatment and continues to manifest the symptoms and signs of hypothyroidism.

Unfortunately, the missed diagnosis of hypothyroidism because of misleading lab results is not the whole story. The Colorado Thyroid Disease Prevalence Study found that when tested for thyroid dysfunction 10% of the study's 25,862 subjects had abnormal findings. That figure, if extended to the general population nationally, would mean there are about 13 million people with undiagnosed thyroid abnormalities. And if, as recommended by many physicians, the upper limit of TSH for thyroid dysfunction were reduced from 5.5 to 3, it would mean that 20% of the population is affected.

Those who have been stressed for long periods of time may have a combination of adrenal fatigue and hypothyroidism. This is because adrenal fatigue can lead to low thyroid production or the thyroid's inability to produce the active type of thyroid. Dr. James Wilson in his book Adrenal Fatigue estimates that 80% of people with low adrenal output will also have low thyroid output. Therefore he stresses, as do a lot of other experts in this field, that it is often advisable to test the adrenals when thyroid pathology exists, and if necessary treat adrenal problems before addressing the thyroid problems.

Clearly, it is not easy to differentiate between hypothyroidism and adrenal fatigue, because one condition can lead to the other. As we have seen, the adrenal gland can play an extensive role on the pituitary, the thyroid gland, and hormones and receptors. And we know that the adrenal gland is affected by stress. But even if the hypothyroid problem is caused by something else (such as an autoimmune disease), the signs and symptoms themselves—fatigue, weight gain, loss of hair, cold and dry skin etcetera—will be a source of stress and will therefore affect the adrenal gland. Vicious cycles are created in any malfunction of the hormonal system and therefore the whole person has to be treated, which means a lifestyle evaluation to identify the root causes, and a stress management regimen in addition to medications and supplement.

CHAPTER 8

How to Kill a Vampire

THE VAMPIRE BATS OF CENTRAL and South America spend their days sleeping, in total darkness, suspended upside down from the roofs of caves. In the dead of night they come out to hunt, alighting on sleeping cows and horses and drink their blood. In a similar way the emotional vampires that are part of the frenetic lives most of us lead suck our vitality and energy. Like the vampire bat they often strike in darkness, their presence undetected, because many times the sources of stress that we experience are so common that we consider them part of a "normal" life. They are not normal for our bodies, however; they are perceived as a threat, and our bodies try to protect us in the only way they know how: by invoking the Stress Response.

The Stress Response evolved to protect us from physical danger, such as wild animals; it was not designed to deal with relationship problems, job pressures, financial pressures, time pressures, and the endless variations on the theme that we face on a daily basis. In the prolonged exposure to those kinds of stressors, as we have seen, it is the Stress Response itself that becomes the threat to our health.

We have no mechanism to automatically protect us from the kinds of stressors we experience today. Since we cannot depend on our bodies to take care of the threat we have to be proactive and develop our own defensive mechanism to counteract the vampire attacks. That defensive mechanism is stress management.

We believe there are five components to an effective stress management program: identifying the sources of stress, and deciding which can be eliminated, changed, or to which we can change our response; adequate nutrition; regular exercise; daily deep relaxation; and medical attention if one has reached the stage of adrenal fatigue.

SOURCES OF STRESS

Often we think we know where our stress is coming from. It may be something obvious, like a parent with Alzheimer's, a teenager on drugs or in trouble with the law, a recent job loss, a divorce, or an abusive boyfriend or girlfriend. Sometimes, often in fact, we do not consciously know all of the vampires that strike in secret. "Stress" has become a word that is part of our everyday lexicon; we use it so often we don't really think any more about what it really means. The four year old daughter of a friend of ours would strike a dramatic pose, close her eyes and strike her forehead with the back of her hand and say: "I'm so stressed!" It was her parents' favorite party entertainment, and of course everyone laughed.

When you begin to seriously address the matter of stress in your life, it can be helpful to use the energy charts we've previously mentioned. We are nourished by many different energy sources—food and water, sources of emotional nourishment, spiritual beliefs and practices—that provide the energy we expend for healing and growth, for movement, for emotional expression, for thought. These are the healthy ways in which we expend energy, but many of us also spend energy in non-productive ways: in worrying, in holding on to negative or painful past experience, bottled up feelings of guilt or regret or resentment, and in the many other ways in which stress impacts our lives. Identifying where our nourishment comes from, and where we spend it, can be a useful first step in taking back control over our own lives. Think of yourself as an energy bank: energy is deposited, and energy is withdrawn. When the withdrawals exceed the deposits, fatigue, lowered immune function, depression, and ultimate systemic breakdown results.

Begin with the Energy Withdrawal chart. Write your name in the center oval, and then fill in the date, so that you will be able to see the changes over time when you refer back to this in the future. Then in the other ovals list all the areas of your life where your energy is going. It doesn't matter whether or not you consider them negative. We all love our children, but we invest enormous resources of energy in caring for them and worrying about them. Notice that stress is any change in the status quo, not just the changes that we perceive as negative. You may want to consider such things as:

People	Situations	Emotions / Habits
Family members (name)	Work / job	Guilt
Friends (name)	Finances	Procrastination
Spouse or ex	Weight	Fear
Social group	Health	Regret
Church group	Unhappy memories	Frustration
Political figures	Survival	Anger
	Education	Feeling victimized
	Relationships	Unworthiness
	Betrayal	Anxiety
		Hopelessness
		Negative self image

Add as many extra ovals as you want. You may want to think about this a while; write everything you can think of and then put it aside and add to it as other things come to mind. When it feels finished assign a number to each oval. These are not percentages, just numbers that intuitively come to mind.

Put this chart away for now, and begin to complete the Energy Deposits chart. You will find that many of the people or situations on the first chart also apply here. For example, children, as mentioned previously, are a huge investment of energy, but they also nurture us in countless ways. Consider such things as:

People	Activities	Emotions
Family	Reading	Satisfaction
Friends	Walking	Things I do well
Co-workers	Exercise	Positive feedback
Pets	Meditating	Accomplishments
Mentors	Church	Freedom
Role Models	Work	Love
	Hobbies	Self-confidence
	Creative projects	Serenity
	Talking to friends	Good health
	Travel	Security
	Study	Humor
	Writing / Journaling	Self-nurture
	Speaking your truth	
	Setting boundaries	

Again, add as many ovals as you want and spend a few days letting the ideas percolate. You may draw a blank when sitting and staring at the page, and then inspiration will strike while you are driving, or when you first wake up, or answer the phone, or take a walk. When the chart feels complete, intuitively assign a number to each oval, and then put the chart aside.

Look at your Ideal Life chart now. Ask yourself the "miracle question." If a miracle happened and you were to wake up tomorrow and find that your life was perfect, what would be the first thing you would notice? What are the component parts of your perfect life? Without considering how it's going to happen, create a chart that contains everything you want your life to contain, including your feelings about yourself.

Now place your three charts side by side. Add up the numbers you assigned to the energy withdrawals and the energy deposits. If your output is greater than your input, you don't have the reserves of energy you need to create your ideal life. The difference between those numbers is what is standing in the way of you creating the life that you want.

Next look at the individual components of the withdrawals chart. Consider the one with the lowest number, which is probably the easiest one to think about changing. What can you do to reduce the amount of energy you are expending on that person, situation or emotion? Let's look at an example.

Teresa's expenditures of energy far outnumbered her deposits, and it was a challenge for her to think about an ideal life. She was so immersed in her suffering that she could not envision many facets of a happy life, and what she did come up with showed that she had what psychologists call an "external locus of control;" she believed that her happiness depended on the actions of others, which left her powerless.

Teresa chose to begin with "missing my father," to which she had assigned a ten, the lowest of her energy expenses. It was too overwhelming at this point to consider her ex-husband, her supervisor or her mother. Teresa did not spend a vast amount of time grieving her father, but thoughts of him still triggered feelings of loss and occasional tears. She recognized, in speaking of him, that her tears were as much about guilt—because she had not told him she loved him—as they were about loss.

Teresa created a special room in her mind, full of her favorite colors and comfortable furniture, and imagined having a conversation with her father, telling him everything she wanted him to know. When she finished, it seemed to her that her father smiled at her and told her how much he loved her and how proud he was of her.

One of the most interesting things about working with imagery is, not only do you get to say the things you did not say in person, but the image answers you. Never, in fifteen years of doing this work, has the image responded with anger, disappointment, or judgment, all the responses we are afraid of.

After her conversation with her father, Teresa found that her thoughts of him no longer evoked feelings of grief and loss; she was able to remember the good times, and thoughts of her father brought feelings of warmth, love, and even laughter as she remembered his sense of humor and the practical jokes he played on his brother. What was a loss on her Energy Withdrawal chart became a gain on her Energy Deposit chart. She found that one small change altered the balance in all areas of her life.

You will find as you work with your energy withdrawals one by one, beginning with the easiest, that there comes a point when everything shifts; you reach a kind of critical mass and it is no longer necessary to tackle each withdrawal individually. Your whole perspective changes and you automatically see everything through a different lens.

Next Teresa considered her Energy Deposits chart. As you can see there were very few areas of her life where she felt nourished. Again, beginning with the smallest number, she began to think about how she could increase her nourishment from that source. "Lunch with women friends" was something that she did only rarely, and only when invited. It was a challenge for her to take the initiative, because she was afraid of rejection, but she made the effort and called her oldest and closest friend, who was delighted to hear from her and eager to see her.

Encouraged by her success, Teresa began to consider the possibility of adding new sources of nourishment. Working from the list of suggestions above, she remembered that she used to love going to church, but she had stopped going after her divorce because she did not want to run into her ex-husband or the people who had known them as a couple. She recognized that she missed the spiritual and social nourishment, but still had the same feelings about going back to her church. She decided to try a new church. It was a giant step for her to go the first time, by herself, but she was welcomed with open arms. Over time she became more active in the church, and ultimately organized a new program for in-home elder care, supervising twenty or more volunteers who visited the homebound.

With these few actions, Teresa made great positive changes in her life and continued to work with her withdrawals. Next, she chose her older sister Karen who bullied her as a child and continued that behavior into adulthood. Again beginning with imagery, Teresa practiced greater assertiveness with Karen and developed a skill that later served her well in confronting her supervisor. Her feelings of loneliness and abandonment took care of themselves as her life filled with activities that offered her companionship and feelings of satisfaction; the feelings of victimization by her ex-husband lessened as she boosted her self esteem and she was able to create stable boundaries in her relationship with her mother.

Karen had relatively few items on each of her charts. You may find your chart crowding itself off the page. The approach is the same: starting with the easiest, you consider the sources of stress—your emotional vampires—one by one. Together, as a group, they may feel overwhelming, but taken one at a time they become manageable.

You will find, as you consider on the Energy Withdrawal Chart the big and little sources of stress in your life, that some of them can be eliminated. If you are someone who has a hard time saying no, for example, and have attracted into your experience one or more emotional vampires who dump their toxic energy on you in long phone conversations full of complaints, you can think about strategies for limiting or eliminating completely their demands on you. You do have the right to say no, and the right—indeed the responsibility—to take care of yourself. If you find when you hang up the phone that you feel drained or tired or depressed, that's a good indicator that the person you've been talking to is an "emotional vampire" for you.

In any uncomfortable situation you have three choices:

- Do nothing and continue to put up with it
- Change the source of the discomfort
- Change your response to it

1. The "do nothing" option.

If you choose the first, of course, nothing will change except you will become more and more worn down.

2. The "change the source" option.

If you choose the second, you can, in the case of the above example, politely but firmly tell the person that you can no longer talk to them, or—if that kind of assertiveness does not feel right, or possible yet—you can think of strategies to limit their demands on you. Practice this response and see if it works for you. Close your eyes and imagine yourself answering the phone; caller ID has alerted you to an acquaintance that typically launches into a litany of complaints. Imagine saying, "Phil. Hi. I only have five minutes I'm afraid." And when four and a half minutes have passed, saying: "I'm so sorry you're having all these difficulties, but I'm going to have to say goodbye. I hope things get better soon."

It might help to remember that offering a sympathetic and ready ear to someone who is a chronic complainer only hurts you and does not help them. They are not looking to change anything; they have developed a habit of looking at the world in a certain way and want you to agree with them. Have you noticed that if you do offer any suggestions for making their situation better they will "yes-but" you to death? We are talking about chronic complainers here; not people you care about who have a specific problem. When you do let them bitch ad nauseum, just about any time they feel like it, you are being an enabler by supporting their complaining habit. It is possible that when you stop offering support, they will realize they can make changes and whether they do or not, it is not your problem.

You can protect yourself from emotional vampires who either leach your energy or dump their toxic energy on you with imagery. Remember, as we saw in Chapter 2, that there is a vast amount of research that supports the effectiveness of imagery in creating positive change, physiologically, emotionally, and in sports performance. For many years now, imagery has been an important part of sports training. Just as imagery is a highly effective tool in sports training, it is highly effective in practicing any kind of response to a challenge, whether that is taking an exam, or being more assertive, or addressing an audience of 500. When you practice a performance in your mind until you can imagine doing it with confidence and comfort, it is easier to perform in the three dimensional world, whether it is the perfect golf swing, or the perfect serve, or saying no to your mother-in-law.

The first time you answer the phone and actually tell Phil you only have five minutes, it might feel like pushing open a door that has been closed for a long time and is stuck, so it takes some effort; then each time you open the door it gets easier and more natural, until you wonder why you ever thought it would be difficult.

Teresa practiced going to a new church many times in her mind before actually doing it, and she found that when she walked through the door it felt familiar instead of something very new and different.

Perhaps one of your emotional vampires is a feeling of helpless anger or resentment over a wrong done to you in the past. The ultimate release of those feelings is through forgiveness, but forgiveness is not always the appropriate first step. When you have been wronged it is important to have the opportunity to speak your truth, to be heard and validated. Speaking your truth to the one who wronged you is not always possible—they may have died, or disappeared—and even if they have not, confrontation is not always the most healing course of action. Survivors of incest who confront their abusers often find that it only creates more suffering. The perpetrator often denies it and makes horrible accusations in turn; other family members don't believe them; the legal system is less than helpful and keeps them locked in the toxic energy of their experience, sometimes for years.

It is just as effective to confront the abuser within the safety of your own mind, in an imaginary place that feels safe to you, with all the imaginary support that you can muster. There you are in complete control and you don't have to deal with any of the backlash that usually happens in a face-to-face confrontation.

When you have an opportunity to express yourself, to say all the things you never had the opportunity to say, then it is time to think about forgiveness. Forgiveness is not saying that what happened is okay; it is simply letting go of feelings that are harmful to you: resentment, anger, helplessness, even revenge. These are toxic emotions that harm only you, not the one who hurt you.

It is possible to do this work on your own, or you may prefer to work with a counselor. Through the Academy for Guided Imagery (www.academyforguidedimagery.com) you can find a counselor certified in Interactive Guided Imagery.

3. The "change your response" option.

The third option is for the situations in which it is not possible, or perhaps not even desirable, to eliminate the stressor from your life. Maybe your boss is driving you up the wall, but you like everything else about your job—it is interesting and challenging, it pays well, the hours work well for you, you get along well with your co-workers, and it's conveniently close—and you really don't want to quit. In this situation, changing your response to the stressor would be the best course of action for you.

Easier said than done, right?

Right. But eminently possible. Again, we begin with imagery, creating a special place in your mind where you can face your boss. Remember that within your own mind you have complete control: you can create any place you want, indoors or out; you decide on the vegetation, the color scheme, the season, the time of day. If your boss intimidates you, give yourself whatever you need in order to feel powerful and safe: a magic cloak, a shield of light, your guardian angel, or your own Samurai.

Perhaps there is so much stored up resentment that you need to vent first and tell your boss exactly what you think of him or her. So go ahead, scream and curse all you want, and when you've got all that out of your system, take a deep breath, surround the angry words in a bubble of light, and blow them away. Venting in the privacy of your own mind will give you relief; venting at your boss may give you temporary relief but is not going to get you to where you want to be. "A soft answer turneth away wrath: but grievous words stir up anger," so says Proverbs. Stirring up his or her anger is not in your best interest, because the boss has more power than you and your goal is to stay at your job.

So there you are, in the safety of the mental sanctuary you have created. You have vented all the wrath and now you turn to the soft approach, speaking your truth clearly and firmly, articulating what you want and imagining him or her responding in the way you want them to respond, saying what you want to hear or at least being open to negotiation.

However disgusted, angry, frustrated, whatever, this person makes you feel, remember that your goal is to make your workplace a pleasant place for you. Your negative emotions fuel the negative atmosphere. Approach this person as you would a stranger, with positive expectations. When you do feel ready to speak to your boss in person, whether or not he or she responds in the way you want you will feel better for having spoken your truth; you will not take personally his or her bad moods; and you will feel strong enough to say "no" to unreasonable demands.

Again, these are procedures that you can use on your own, with the help of a pencil and paper and CDs. You may prefer to work with a professional such as a counselor or minister, but be sure to find someone with whom you feel comfortable, whom you can trust, who has your best interests at heart and is not going to support an agenda that includes reinforcing specific roles. Some Christian counselors or ministers, for example, perceive their role as reinforcing traditional Christian values, which are not always the same as helping you to reclaim your own power.

NUTRITION

The second component of an effective stress management program is adequate nutrition. You can be doing everything else right, but if you are not receiving the right kind of nourishment, your body will be stressed.

As important as what you eat, and the amount you eat, is how you eat. Long gone, for most of us, are the three daily meals prepared by mom and the evening family meal seated around the table. Breakfast, for many of us, is a cup of coffee and maybe some kind of starchy, sugary pastry. Lunch might be a sandwich or a hamburger from the drive-up window of a fast food restaurant, eaten in the car while driving and listening to the radio/talking on the phone/texting at red lights. Dinner is often in front of the TV.

When we eat while doing something else, in a hurry, the mind full of tumbling thoughts, we are eating while under stress. As we know, one of the effects of the stress response is to shut-down non essential systems. The stress response slows the digestive process, because digesting is not a priority when life is in danger. A stress-filled life means we suffer various illnesses of the digestive tract: acid reflux, indigestion, constipation or diarrhea, heartburn. Good news for the pharmaceutical companies but not so good for our well-being.

Many years ago, after attending a conference in San Diego, we were scheduled to fly out of Los Angeles and needed to find a hotel to spend the night. In a used bookstore, down a side street somewhere in San Diego, we found an old guidebook with a description of a newly built Japanese hotel with a rooftop Shinto garden.

When we arrived, we discovered that the "newly built" hotel was now a couple of decades old and had become the heart of a kind of little Tokyo. It did indeed have a beautiful roof top garden, and the restaurant was alongside with a wall of windows giving the illusion of being outdoors. The classic Japanese décor was of pure clean lines and the "waitress" an exquisite vision in a kimono who seemed to glide as if on invisible roller skates. She served us a traditional

Japanese breakfast of tasty morsels served in beautiful lacquered bowls. The only sound was the falling water and a distant shamisen. The only other patrons at that early hour were a couple of Japanese businessmen in three-piece suits. We all ate in silence, focusing on the delicate flavors of the food and the visual feast of the garden. And we thought: Sure, we can face LAX after starting the day out this way.

Whenever possible, try to eat in a relaxed atmosphere, and chew slowly, allowing yourself to thoroughly enjoy all the tastes and textures. Why? Because digestion begins in the mouth. Food hurriedly chewed and swallowed in chunks never becomes fully digested, and we lose the benefit of much of the nutrition it contains, even if it is organic and well balanced.

Saying grace before meals is a quaint, old-fashioned concept for most of us and yet cultivating an attitude of gratitude is one of the easiest and most powerful ways of creating a shift towards feelings of well-being, including improving digestion. One of the exercises offered by mindful meditation is to eat a raisin, fully mindful of every aspect of its existence: the grape on the vine, the sun on the grape, the rain, the one who harvested it, the drying process; and the look of it, how it feels resting in your palm, the feel of it on your tongue, and so on. When you do this exercise you can spend ten or fifteen minutes eating a single raisin.

Of course, we are talking about food as nourishment, not eating as meditation, but bringing awareness to the activity of eating helps in cultivating an attitude of appreciation and slows the process of eating so that all the body's digestive functions work efficiently. If you try to eat at least one meal a day in a relaxed atmosphere, allowing time to be thankful, aware of the colors, shapes and textures of the food, you will soon notice a difference in your physical, mental and emotional well-being.

What do you eat as part of a stress management program?

A healthy stress management diet is one that provides all the essential nutrients the body needs, roughage for good digestion and elimination, and only the number of calories the body needs to maintain its ideal weight and size. It is made up of a balance between protein, complex carbohydrates, and good fats.

Proteins provide the basic building blocks to build healthy tissue. They are found in lean meats, legumes, tofu, eggs, nuts and dairy products. A good rule of thumb is that protein should be one third of the volume of food on your plate, and be about the size of a pack of cards, less if you are using nuts as a protein source because they are high in fat.

Complex carbohydrates (the good carbs) are in vegetables, fruits, and whole grains. Reading labels is a must here: many breads claiming to be whole wheat contain mostly white flour and only some whole wheat, sometimes as little as a tablespoon, and many contain refined sugar. Complex carbs should make up the other two thirds of food on your plate, though green, orange and red vegetables can be eaten in abundance. Without gobs of fatty dressing, naturally.

Simple carbohydrates (the bad carbs) are pretty much anything white: refined flour, refined sugar, white rice, potatoes without skins. They cause the blood sugar to go on a roller coaster ride, causing fluctuating energy levels and cravings for more refined carbs. They should be eaten sparingly or avoided altogether. Don't forget about the sugar in wine, beer and soft drinks.

Good fats are unsaturated fats. Sunflower, sesame, safflower, corn, and flax seed oil are high in the essential Omega-6 and Omega-3 fatty acids. These fats are called "essential" because the body does not make them. Olive oil and coconut oils are probably the healthiest. Fatty acids are good sources of energy and are an essential part of the body's oxygen transport mechanism as well as key building blocks of the cells and hormones. The subject of fats in diets is complicated and a book on its own. Fortunately there are many books on fats, unfortunately there are many opinions. Important is that omega 3 fatty acids should trump the intake over omega 6 fatty acids since the latter detract from the body's use of the more important omega 3.

Most of us obtain ample amounts of Omega-6 fatty acids from our regular diet, but are deficient in the Omega-3 fatty acids. These are found in certain fish, such as mackerel, sardines, tuna, trout, and cold-water salmon, and are also available in capsule form from health food stores. Flax seed oil is a good source of Omega-3 for vegetarians who choose not to take fish oils. You can buy it cold pressed but it's very expensive and needs to be refrigerated. It is much less expensive and just as effective to buy flax seeds and grind them in a coffee grinder. You can grind quite a lot to freeze for later use. Add it to cereals or protein shakes.

Bad fats are the saturated fats, found in fatty meats, whole milk products, and oils that have been refined or treated to make them solid, e.g. margarine and vegetable shortening. The heating process changes the molecular structure of the oil and changes it from a good fat into a trans fatty acid, the worst kind of fat. These are the fats that clog arteries and contribute to heart disease and circulatory problems.

It would be best to eat a balance of protein, complex carbohydrates and healthy fat at every meal, including snacks. The body metabolizes these food groups at different rates: first the complex carbs, then the protein, then the fats. This maintains a steady blood sugar level for about three hours and avoids the sugar highs and lows discussed in Chapter 5, not only keeping your mood on even keel but also avoiding the cravings for inappropriate foods that upset the sugar balance—and therefore your mood—and pile on the unwanted fat.

What about dairy? Cow's milk is very good—for baby cows. The molecular structure of cow's milk is not appropriate for many of us and can cause problems with the digestive system, and as with meats the hormones and antibiotics fed to cows find their way into the milk. But many of us who are convinced of the benefits of a dairy free diet are still loathe to abandon favorite cheeses and milk.

Soy, rice and almond milk can be substituted for cow's milk, but don't expect any of them to taste like milk. Be sure that they are not genetically modified and are organic; rice should not be grown in soil containing arsenic. If you approach them as a new food without any particular expectations you may find that you actually like them. Almond and rice milk are sweeter than soy and lower in protein. Try a few different brands—it's all a matter of preference. Most are organic, but check the label to be sure. By all means eat your favorite cheese once in a while, or flavor your vegetables with a teaspoon of butter (preferably organic, from cows not fed hormones or antibiotics), though after a while of experiencing a dairy free diet you may find you don't miss it as much.

There are cheeses available made from soy or rice protein that taste something like the real thing. They are more successful, I think, in cooked foods such as eggplant parmesan than eaten simply as cheese. Cubed in salads or sliced in sandwiches with other ingredients they can add flavor, and as a bonus they are much lower in calories than regular cheese.

A final word about sugar; most of us are habituated to excess sweetness. Sugar is added to many commercial food products, such as breads, canned vegetables, and canned fruits that float in a highly concentrated sugar goo, and most prepared foods. Soft drinks contain up to ten teaspoons of refined sugar. Even our cakes, desserts, and pies contain much more sugar than similar foods in other countries.

Refined sugar is a simple carbohydrate that is absorbed quickly into the bloodstream causing a sugar high. When the blood sugar level drops, there is a loss of energy and craving for more sugar. Dietary sugar is a contributor to the current high incidence of Diabetes type II, as we saw in Chapter 5.

If you choose to cut down on your sugar intake it may take a while to accustom yourself to a lower level of sweetness, but when you do you will find a whole range of new flavors to enjoy. Substituting synthetic sweeteners is not s a good idea; some are known carcinogens, others may prove to be, and if you continue to feed a sweetness craving it only leads to more craving and a probable return at some point to refined sugar.

Preferred sweeteners, those that still contain their natural vitamins and trace minerals, are Succinate, honey, agave juice and organic maple syrup. You can also try dried granulated dates, available at health food stores. But a more desirable goal is to re-educate your palate to enjoy a lower level of sweetness.

Alcohol and nicotine—we don't have to remind anybody, do we?—are poisons best eliminated. Drink alcohol in moderation. Nicotine is a no-no.

If you are a ten-cup-a-day coffee addict, type A driven personality constantly on the go who skips meals, or a busy working mother who's survival depends on fast foods, or any one of the infinite varieties on those themes, you are obviously not going to change everything about your diet overnight. But, if you are at least persuaded of the desirability of making changes, you can begin slowly, perhaps by promising yourself a healthy balanced breakfast. Remember, one-third protein to two-thirds complex carbohydrates, which is obviously not eggs and bacon and home fries. A slice of whole grain toast with a poached or scrambled egg and fruit? A half-cup of non-fat cottage cheese and a banana? Low or non-fat yogurt with Muesli? Once you notice the benefits of making these changes, it will become easier and easier. Remember to think about a healthy diet as being a matter of self nurture, not self denial.

EXERCISE

The Stress Response prepares the body for physical action—to fight or to flee—so exercise is a highly effective stress management tool because it provides the physical exertion that gives the body the signal to return to its normal resting state. And, as a bonus, exercise has been shown to be as effective as anti-depressants for mild to moderate depression. Unlike the SSRI antidepressants, it has only positive side effects: toned muscles that are not easily injured and recover more quickly when they are injured; glowing skin; strong bones; a trim and energetic body that feels good to you and looks good to others; more energy and vitality; greater strength; clarity of mind and focus; and . . . we think we've made the point.

The best exercise is one that combines resistance (weight training) with flexibility and endurance (for the cardiovascular and respiratory systems.) Yoga will give you all three, as well as deep relaxation and deep breathing, and many yoga classes include meditation. There are many different schools of Yoga teaching different kinds of Yoga and it is best to begin with a qualified teacher. But, as mentioned in Chapter 6, there are innumerable choices of exercise options available. Aim for at least thirty minutes, five times a week.

The exercise that is best for you is the one you enjoy and, therefore, will do. Even a short walk three times a week is better than nothing. Again, begin slowly if exercise is not yet a part of your life. Recruit a friend to walk with you if you like company and can benefit from reinforcement. If you are a parent, you can make family walks part of your time together, which has the added benefit of teaching healthy habits to your children. Refer back to Chapter 6 for more suggestions on beginning an exercise program.

RELAXATION

When was the last time you really, truly, relaxed? Many of us don't even remember what it feels like. Make a fist with your right hand and squeeze as hard as you can. Now let it go. It's obvious that it take a lot of energy to do that, and yet many of us walk around holding that level of tension all the time, in our shoulders, lower back, stomach. Such tension interferes with restful sleep, gives us tension headaches, digestive problems, high blood pressure, as well as all the hormonal imbalances discussed throughout this book.

As a society we spend billions of dollars a year on medications to reduce blood pressure, tension headaches, anxiety, and to help us to sleep. We have been conditioned by geniuses of manipulation in the advertising industry to believe that there is a pill for every discomfort, an easy solution to each of life's challenges.

However, all medications have potential negative side effects and many of them are habit forming. Medications for blood pressure can adversely affect the liver; anxiety medications can cause decreased concentration, memory impairment and impaired cognitive functioning; high doses of sedatives can impair respiration and blood pressure. In spite of these risks we have been persuaded to prefer the medical solution, and we are resistant to the idea that lifestyle changes can have the same or better psychological and physiological benefits as medication.

We saw in Chapter 2 that the benefits of guided imagery, progressive muscle relaxation, yoga, t'ai chi and meditation have been extensively researched and proven beneficial as part of a stress management program. Learning the Relaxation Response and allowing yourself a daily relaxation practice of as little as twenty or thirty minutes is a natural, healthy, cost effective, simple and highly effective tool within reach of everyone to counteract the effects of the stressors that we all live with. The benefits are immense: health, vitality, better sleep, increased immune function, greater concentration, focus and productivity, and an all-around increased sense of well-being. If you think you don't have the time, consider this: the average American spends over four hours a day watching television.

As with exercise, the form of relaxation that works best for you is the one you enjoy. For some, it's a weekly yoga class and daily practice at home; it can be a warm bath, spiced up with candles and soft music; it can be a massage, (though you're unlikely to do that every day, unless you and your partner massage each other. Even a ten minute foot massage or head massage can be wonderfully relaxing); it can be a walk by yourself; you can learn self hypnosis and put yourself into a deep trance for ten or fifteen minutes a day; you can listen to a CD of guided imagery; you can take a meditation class and practice daily at home.

Even as little as ten or fifteen minutes a day can make a huge difference. As you learn and practice the Relaxation Response, you are inducing the opposite reactions of the Stress Response, allowing your body to settle down into a healthy, resting state. Here is a comparison of the physiological effects of the Stress Response (SR) and the Relaxation Response (RR):

Under the SR, the heart rate and the force of contraction of the heart increase to provide blood to the heart, lungs, brain and large muscles. During the RR the heart rate is reduced, blood pressure is reduced.

SR: blood is shunted away from the skin and internal organs, except the heart and lungs.

RR: Blood is shunted towards internal organs, especially those involved in digestion.

SR: The rate of breathing increases to supply oxygen to the heart, brain, and exercising muscle.

RR: Rate of breathing decreases as oxygen demand is reduced during periods of rest.

SR: Increased sweat to eliminate toxins and lower body temperature.

RR: sweat decreases.

SR: Production of digestive juices is severely reduced.

RR: production of digestive juices increases, improving digestion.

SR: Blood sugar levels are dramatically increased as the liver dumps stored glucose into the bloodstream.

RR: blood sugar levels are maintained in the normal range.

The more you practice the Relaxation Response, the more you will take the feeling of calm into your daily life, no matter where you are, what you are doing, or what is going on around you.

Again, implementing the components of an effective stress management program is not going to happen overnight. What can happen overnight is that you make a start. Choose any one of these areas—insight, diet, exercise, relaxation—and make a promise to yourself to be consistent with at least one element for at least one month. The difference in the way you feel—physically, emotionally and mentally—will be your incentive to continue.

Medical attention

If after an extended period of chronic stress you have reached the stage of adrenal fatigue, please seek medical attention, preferably from an holistic physician who will be able to combine the best of allopathic and alternative treatments to support your adrenals and bring your hormones back into balance, as you do your part by implementing the other four components of your new, managed stress lifestyle.

Killing vampires is not easy. It takes commitment and practice in establishing a new way of thinking, feeling, and doing until it feels natural. Remember that there are no failures except the failure of not trying. And if you backslide, it's no great tragedy; just pick up where you left off and recognize the small steps of progress. It took a long time to practice living with stress; so be gentle with yourself and give yourself time to change directions.

CHAPTER 9

Some Final Words

THE TRANSYLVANIAN VAMPIRES OF LEGEND suck the blood of their victims and cause physical and psychological changes that turn them into monsters.

The myriad emotional vampires that are part and parcel of the frenetic lives most of us lead suck our vitality and energy. Our bodies perceive the threat and try to protect us in the only way they know how, by invoking the Stress Response. But the Stress Response evolved to protect us from physical danger, such as wild animals, which required that we fight or run. It was not designed to deal with demanding jobs, busy family schedules, or the in-laws, for example and in the prolonged exposure to those kinds of stressors, it is the stress response itself that becomes the threat to our health. We have no mechanism to automatically protect us from the kinds of stressors we experience today. We cannot depend on our bodies to take care of the threat; we have to take charge and develop our own defensive mechanism: stress management.

Emotional vampires may be the root cause of almost all hormonal problems. Stress causes the adrenal glands to produce cortisol; chronic stress causes the adrenals to continue to produce cortisol until the gland is run down, the condition known as adrenal fatigue. Our bodies were not designed to cope with chronic stress, but only with immediate and short-lived stress.

The Stress Response prepares the body to fight or to run, the appropriate response to the kinds of stressors we encountered when Homo sapiens evolved. Cortisol production is nature's way of producing a "flight or fight" response that should last only for a short time, a burst of energy that allows us to flee from a tiger or fight the group trying to steal the women or the food. The burst of physical activity signals the adrenals to stop producing cortisol, and the body's systems return to their normal resting state.

When the stress is chronic, as so many of modern day stresses are, it presents a whole different pathological problem. When cortisol is constantly produced it becomes known as the "death hormone," because it decreases or completely eliminates the hormones of aldosterone (which regulates blood pressure), estrogen, progesterone, testosterone and thyroid. Why? Because these hormones are not necessary for the flight or fight response.

And therein lies the beginning of a multitude of problems. The solution is to address the cause of the problem and learn stress management. We often hear from patients that they know where their stress is coming from, but on further investigation it almost always comes out that there are multiple sources or that the main stressor is not what they thought it was. They often say that they can't do anything to change it, and perhaps that is true, but they can change how they respond to and cope with the stressor. And they can make lifestyle changes that will manage the effects of stress by following the steps outlined in the previous chapter.

We were not created to be driven, worried, harried, uptight, fearful, and tense. We were created to express the joy of life. In our busy lives focused on doing, we often forget that we are human beings. It is enough to be; to stop and smell the roses; to live fully in the now and cherish and relish each moment to the fullest, instead of allowing life to pass us by while we focus on the tasks of everyday life. I hope if nothing else that the information in this book has encouraged you to remember that you are a unique and wonderful individual, deserving of respect and self-love and self nurture. I hope you will take the first steps towards restructuring your life to make time for nurturing all aspects of your being: physical, emotional, mental and spiritual. It is your birthright. Please claim it.

APPENDICES

APPENDIX I

Synopsis of Functions of the Hormones

I. Cortisol

At healthy levels, cortisol influences, regulates, and moderates:

- Blood sugar levels
- Fat, protein, and carbohydrate metabolism
- Immune responses
- Anti-inflammatory mechanisms
- Blood pressure
- The central nervous system

Elevated cortisol levels cause:

- Impaired cognitive functioning
- Low thyroid and eventual hypothyroidism
- Decreased bone density
- Insomnia
- Decreased muscle mass
- Elevated blood pressure
- Slower wound healing

- Increased fat deposits, especially around the abdominal area, which can contribute to cardiovascular problems.

Low cortisol levels cause:

- Foggy brain
- Depression
- Low blood sugar or hypoglycemia
- Fatigue
- Insomnia
- Low blood pressure
- Decreased immune function
- Increased inflammation

II. Estrogen

Estrogen is responsible for:

- Female secondary sex characteristics such as breast growth and female hair pattern.
- Stimulates osteoblast (bone cell) activity, increasing bone growth and strength
- Promotes moderate protein enhancement
- Deposition of subcutaneous fat
- Promotes soft and smooth skin texture
- Sodium and water retention
- Prevents "brain fog"
- Sexual feelings and emotional stability
- Counteracts excessive levels of progesterone and protects the female organs

Decreased estrogen levels lead to:

- Anxiety
- Dry skin
- Loss of libido and orgasms
- Memory loss
- Vaginal dryness
- Yeast infections
- Depression
- Headaches
- Hot flashes
- Mood swings
- Night sweats
- Painful intercourse
- Insomnia
- Palpitations

III. Progesterone

Progesterone is responsible for:

- Preparation of the uterus for pregnancy
- Breast preparation for lactation
- Protects against estrogen dominance
- Required for successful pregnancies
- Helps form the myelin sheath around neurons of the brain
- Prevents water retention
- Contributes to new bone growth
- Reduces cravings for carbohydrates
- Raises thyroid hormone level and therefore helps breakdown fat and reduce hair loss
- Anti-anxiety

Progesterone deficiency signs and symptoms:

- Anxiety
- Cramps
- Headache
- Menstrual problems
- Insomnia
- Low libido
- Painful and/or swollen breasts
- Bloating
- Depression
- Fuzzy thinking
- Food Cravings
- Moodiness
- Weight gain

IV. Testosterone

At healthy levels is responsible for:

- Muscle and bone growth and strength
- Brain and heart protection in males and females
- Libido and erections
- Incentive in business and everyday happenings
- Enhances male and female cognition
- Helps prevent and slow Alzheimer's Disease
- Produces more nitric oxide which dilates blood vessels
- Improves cellular oxygen levels
- Prevention of andropause
- Some studies show benefit to diabetic alleviation and arthritis alleviation
- Helps control blood sugar and cholesterol
- Male physical traits
- Antidepressant in males and females

For signs of testosterone deficiency, see Appendix IV

V. Thyroid

Needed to metabolize food and produce energy and heat.
A deficiency is hypothyroidism, which causes weight gain.
Over production is hyperthyroidism, which causes weight loss.

Hypothyroid symptoms:

- Constipation
- Fatigue
- Hair loss and loss of lateral 1/3 of eyebrows
- Low energy
- Weight gain with increase in cholesterol and triglyceride levels
- Cold intolerance with body temperature below 97.7 or 97.4
- Cold hands and feet
- Incentive loss
- Skin is dry and scaly and hair and nails are brittle and dry. Skin is often thick and dry especially over the shins. This is called myxedema
- Increased capillary permeability and, therefore, edema
- Muscular weakness and joint stiffness and slow tendon reflexes
- Depression

Perimenopausal and menopausal women often have hypothyroidism which is often overlooked by the physician

VI. Aldosterone

- Promotes transport of sodium and potassium via the kidneys and thereby keeps these mineral ions in balance.

- Low aldosterone levels lead to decreased levels of sodium; while at the same time a potassium increase via the urine. The opposite is also true.
- An increase of sodium leads to an increase of water retention and therefore an increase in blood pressure. "Where ever sodium goes, so follows water." (James Wilson, ND, PhD, DC)
- Excessive loss of potassium (hypokalemia) prevents normal nerve and muscle electrical impulses causing muscle weakness.
- High potassium causes cardiac toxicity with dysrhythmias and eventual death.
- Aldosterone causes absorption of sodium from the intestines and colon. Therefore aldosterone failure causes loss of sodium chloride and water and diarrhea.
- Keeps magnesium and chloride balance
- Hydrates tissues and cells.
- Maintains the blood volume.
- Salt cravings occur with low aldosterone.

VII.   DHEA

- DHEA is produced by the same part of the adrenal as cortisol and can be measured at the same time as cortisol levels using sputum testing.
- Precursor for several hormones.
- The adrenals cannot produce DHEA and cortisol at the same time; therefore, when cortisol is high the DHEA will be low or none.
- Some women do not do well on DHEA due to side effects such as facial hair and acne, which are androgenic effects. The alternative is to use either progesterone or pregenenolone. These are both made from cholesterol. Both of these can be converted into other hormones. Pregenenolone is a precursor

to androstanededion, which can be converted to testosterone or Estradiol or estrone.

- The most abundant hormone produced by the adrenals and the most abundant hormone in the blood stream under normal conditions in the form of DHEA-S.
- Because cortisol is, in general, a catabolic (breaking down) hormone, the antagonist needed is an anabolic (building up) hormone. This is DHEA. Therefore, testing for DHEA-S and finding it low is often an early warning that the adrenal glands are failing.

Hormones and their Interactions

Hormones and their Interactions

Anabolic Hormone = A Building Hormone DHEA	Catabolic Hormone = A Dismantling Hormone DHT

STRESS → CORTISOL ⚖ at First ————————————→ Androstendione
    When stress continues, the   (→ ⚖ Testosterone)
    adrenal wears out and one has   Progesterone
    little or no Cortisol output. This is   Estrogen
    Adrenal Fatigue.   Aldosterone
                                     Thyroid   Estrone
                                     DHEA   ↕
                                                  Estradiol

CHOLESTEROL → Pregnenolone → DHEA → Androstendione → Testosterone
With the intervening   ↘   ↗ Aldosterone   ↘
help of Aldosterone   Progesterone   DHT
and Potassium   ↘ Cortisol

ESTROGEN ———→ ⚖ Insulin + ⚖ Androgens → ♣ ⚖ FAT
(and Birth Control Pills)   (Testosterone)
                  ⚖ Prolactin + ⚖ Testosterone → ♣ ⚖ FAT

         SHGB ————————→ Testosterone → ♣ ⚖ FAT
        (Sex Hormone
        Binding Globulin)

     FAT Itself ————→ SHGB → ♣ ⚖ FAT

SEROTONIN ————→ ⚖ Prolactin + ⚖ Testosterone → ♣ ⚖ FAT
(SSRI Drugs)

♣ = Therefore

Appendix III

Clinical tests for adrenal fatigue

- Blood pressure decrease of more than 10mm/hg when going from a supine to upright position.
- The pupils cannot hold contraction when light is shone in eyes.
- Sergant's sign: a line drawn on the abdomen remains whitish in color instead of turning red.
- Rogoff's sign: pain or tenderness over the adrenals when pressed. The adrenals are found below the posterior 12th rib. Pressure is applied with the thumbs as the patient breaths in and out
- The thyroid should be tested as well as thyroid dysfunction and adrenal fatigue often occur together, or thyroid dysfunction alone can manifest with very similar symptoms.
- Saliva cortisol/DHEA testing.

Appendix IV

Signs and Symptoms of Menopause and Andropause

Menopause	Andropause
Anxiety	Anxiety
Irritability	Irritability
Fatigue	Fatigue
Loss of energy	Loss of energy
Poor concentration	Poor concentration
Depression	Depression
Loss of muscle tone	Loss of muscle tone
Decreased exercise tolerance	Decreased exercise tolerance
Prolonged recovery from exercise	Prolonged recovery from exercise
Little or no improvement with exercise	Little or no improvement with exercise
Weight gain in spite of exercise	Weight gain in spite of exercise
Loss of memory	Loss of memory
Osteoporosis	Osteoporosis
Decreased sexual desire	Decreased sexual desire
Cardiac disease	Cardiac disease
Higher bad cholesterol	Higher bad cholesterol
Hot flashes	Hot flashes (some men)
Night sweats	Night sweats (some men)
	Prostate enlargement

Like any other hormone deficiency—such as thyroid, insulin, or estrogen-progesterone—deficient testosterone in men or women will interfere with a healthy and vigorous life and contribute to aging. Natural, bio-identical testosterone is available but is often avoided because of misunderstandings and myths about the role of this vital hormone.

Testosterone earned a bad rep from publicity of its abuse by athletes. However, the testosterone that the athletes were using was synthetic and it was used in enormous quantities. The body does not know what to do with synthetic chemicals whose molecular structures are different from the structure of substances produced naturally by the body. As with any medicine, natural or pharmaceutical, the dose must be appropriate and therefore individualized to the person.

A lot of men do not understand why symptoms and signs occur as they age, such as weight gain in spite of exercise and larger, flaccid breasts. Depression, irritability, mood swings, loss of morning erections, erectile dysfunction, poor focus and concentration, loss of initiative in things they once enjoyed and business, loss of muscle tone and night sweats. All of the above are probably what is termed "andropause" or more easily understood as male menopause.

Men produce lower levels of testosterone with age. This decline in testosterone production starts at about 30—35 years of age and lasts until the ages of 50—60. The effects of lowered testosterone are subtle in contrast to the effects of menopause, which in most women lasts from 1 to 8 years.

Most people think of testosterone just as the hormone that annoys women. So much academic work has been done demonstrating the remarkable role testosterone plays in men and women.

Testosterone is the main muscle and bone building hormone. It is not just calcium, vitamin K, and vitamin D, and boron that build bones—it is testosterone. For women, estrogen and progesterone certainly help but it is testosterone that is the primary bone builder. I believe it is a lot safer than Fosamax and Actonel. This is why men do not get osteoporosis until a much later age then women. But if we do get osteoporosis and break a hip, we have 30% chance of dying from an embolus as compared to a women having a 9% chance of dying. Unfortunately, doctors often do not test men for osteoporosis thinking it is a women's problem.

Evidence shows there are 3—4 times more testosterone receptors on the heart cells than in the gonads, implying that testosterone protects the heart. Testosterone also helps produce nitric oxide, which is like taking synthetic nitroglycerine to expand the vessels and give better circulation.

Testosterone receptors are also present in the brain. Using Functional MRI (fMRI), which shows the part of the brain that is performing a specific function, it was shown that men and women with low testosterone levels were more "foggy brained." In fact, when levels were really low they could not fantasize. This is evidence, as noted on fMRI, that there are testosterone receptors in the brain. Other studies have shown that lower testosterone levels correlate with increased occurrence of Alzheimer's disease. Giving testosterone to men with Alzheimer's slowed disease progression significantly, although it did not cure it. This also demonstrates the presence of testosterone receptors in the brain.

It is now known that 60—70% of depression in men over 50 could be secondary to low testosterone levels. I can attest to this myself. The use of toxic antidepressants could be avoided with the proper testosterone replacement.

Testing for testosterone levels is simple, requiring only blood samples. It is wise to perform testing for more than just testosterone, however. One needs to know the total testosterone and also the amount available to get into the cells. The latter is called free testosterone because testosterone can bind to a protein called the Sex hormone binding protein (SHBG). If testosterone is not bound to SHBG, it is "free." One can have high testosterone levels, but if it is not getting into the cells, meaning there is not enough free testosterone available, it does no good. Next, a man also needs to know his estrogen level (estradiol) because testosterone normally converts to estrogen. This conversion of testosterone to estrogen is called aromatization and is accomplished by the aromatase enzyme. The aromatase enzyme is found in adipose tissue, also called fatty tissue. This explains why, as men age and body fat increases, there is an increase in conversion of testosterone to estrogen. The more estrogen produced, the more fat is produced due to estrogen effect. Estrogen also stimulates more production of SHBG. It is a vicious cycle. The physician needs to be aware of the interplay amongst these hormones so as to not inadvertently cause more andropause symptoms. Aromatization can be blocked, so no need to worry.

Blood tests are worthless unless interpreted properly, as described above, and accompanied by a thorough interview with a physician who, hopefully, thinks outside the box. Why? Because if the blood tests come back in the low normal range, the physician will likely say, "Oh, your level of testosterone is normal." Yes, but normal for an eighty year old! Who wants to feel like an eighty year old? The symptoms and signs are just as important as correct interpretation of blood tests. A proper assessment is only achieved with a thorough history and physical, which will take about an hour. Other blood tests may be warranted, depending on the interview, especially a Prostate Specific Antigen (PSA) test to rule out a prostate problem.

The belief that testosterone causes cancer of the prostate is a myth. I was taught this 40 years ago in medical school. If it were true, men at twenty years old, when the testosterone is the highest, would have prostate cancer. It is now known that estrogen causes prostate cancer—the same hormone that causes women to have breast and uterine cancer. This is because there is a vestige of the uterus inside the prostate, called a utricle, which has estrogen receptors. It is still uncertain if a man currently has prostate cancer whether testosterone will speed up its growth because testosterone is a growth hormone but not the cause of he cancer.

There are a few ways to take testosterone, but one should always use bio-identical natural hormones, which are exact duplicates of what one's body would make if it were still able. Bio-identical hormones are usually made from soy and must be compounded by a compounding pharmacist, often to the exact specifications of the patient. They are not available at a big chain pharmacy. I prefer topical hormone creams and pellets. Hormone pellets are inserted, by the physician, under the skin of the buttocks. I do not use oral testosterone because levels fluctuate and can be harmful to the liver.

There are pros and cons with both methods of administering testosterone. Creams must be applied once or twice a day, which the patient must remember to do. There can be a roller coaster effect depending on the person's skin and absorption and their chemical make-up. Also if one is traveling they need to remember to take the cream with them. Creams work well and are absorbed in about twenty minutes.

Pellets are bio-identical hormones in solid form, of about the size of a grain of rice, and are inserted under the skin of the buttocks with local anesthesia. They last about 5-6 months depending on the activity of the person because increased pumping of the heart and the resultant increased blood flow will hasten absorption of the pellet. When the person is sedentary, the heart pumps the blood slower and the pellet absorbs much more slowly. There is no roller coaster effect with the pellets and one does not have to be concerned about remembering to take them.

I usually like to start off with creams, assess the effectiveness for the individual and redo blood tests, including PSA, in about 6—8 weeks. I can then discuss pellets as an option if the patient has a preference or their condition warrants.

One does get older, but one does not have to age. It is not only longevity but also quality of longevity. I hope this introduction has helped you.

APPENDIX V

Tests Warranted Before and After HRT

I-Males pre-hormone replacement

- Complete Blood Count [CBC]
- Comprehensive Metabolic Panel—especially since it has the liver functions.
- Cholesterol including HDL, LDL, Triglycerides, and a cardiac heart ratio.
- PSA [prostate specific antigen] for testing the prostate. Not a great test but all we have in the way of blood tests to screen for cancer of the prostate. It is important to know the difference in change even if a previous PSA was normal and the latest one is normal. If there is big difference then further follow up should be considered.
- Estradiol: it is important to know this level before testosterone therapy to check latter on if the testosterone is converting to estrogen.
- Testosterone—free and total
- SHBG if your physician believes in it at this time. Some wait and get it if the man is not doing as well as predicted.
- Any other tests if the client has specific problems. This is especially true for liver function tests [LFT] if the history

suggests this should be done; for example if the client is a heavy drinker.

II-Males after 2-4 months recheck when on bio-identical testosterone

- Testosterone free and total
- Estradiol
- PSA
- SHBG if physician feels it necessary
- Liver function tests if physician feels it necessary from the history.
- DHT [dihydrotestosterone] if there seems to be a problem that would relate to testosterone converting too much to this strong type of testosterone.

III-Females pre—hormone replacement

- CBC [complete blood count]
- Comprehensive Metabolic Panel, especially for the liver enzymes
- Estradiol
- Testosterone free and total
- Some doctors like a sonogram of the uterus to check for fibroids and any abnormalities of the uterus.
- Any other exams pertinent to the patient after a history and physical
- Follicle Stimulating Hormone [FSH]
- I like to check the thyroid lab at this time since perimenopause and menopause so often go together. If not the whole thyroid panel then at least TSH [Thyroid Stimulating Hormone].

IV—Females after 2-4 months recheck

- Testosterone free and total
- Estradiol
- SHBG if considered necessary by physician
- Any additional tests needed for medical reasons.
- Further thyroid testing if signs and symptoms and labs indicate it is necessary. This may include thyroid testing to see if the person has an autoimmune disease for low thyroid.

BIBLIOGRAPHY

Baron, S. H. "An Investigation of Absorptive Ca[acity in the Efficacy of Imagery Training in Performance of an Instep Kick by selected Youth Soccer Players." *Dissertation Abstracts International: Section B: The Sciences and Engineering,* 61(2000): 2265. Accessed February 10, 2007 from the EbscoHOST database.

Boyd, E. S., M.D. & M. Konneg PhD. "Paleolithic Nutrition." *New England Journal of Medicine.* 312(1985): 283-289.

Burns, D. S. "The Effect of the Bonny Method of Guided Imagery and Music Quality of Life and Cortisol Levels of Cancer Patients." *Dissertation Abstracts International Section A: Humanities and Social Sciences,* 61(2000): 20. Accessed February 1, 2007 from the EbscoHOST database.

Cousins, Norman *Anatomy of an Illness.* New York: Bantam Books, 1979.

Fox, H. C., Talih, M., Malison, R., Anderson, G. M., Kreek, M. J. & Sinha, R. "Frequency of Recent Cocain and Alcohol Use Affects Drug Craving and Associated Responses to Stress and Drug-Related Cues." *Psychoneuroendocrinology* 30(2009).

Fox, H. C., Garcia, M., Kemp, K., Milivojevic V., Kreek, M. J & Sinha, R. "Gender Differences in Cardiovascular and Corticoadrenal

Response to stress and Cues in Cocaine Dependent Individuals."
Psychopharmacology 185(2006): 348-357. Accessed February 1,
2007, from the EbscoHOST database.

Genazzani, A. R. et al. "Adrenal Function Under Long-Term
Raloxifene Administration." *Gynecology Endocrinology*
17(2003):159-168.

Graveline, D., MD. *Lipitor, Thief of Memory.* Duane Graveline, MD,
2006.

Hanrahan, C. (1995). "In Search of a 'Good' Image: Use of Imagery
While Performing Dance Movement." *Dissertation Abstracts
International Section A: Humanities and Social Sciences* 55(1995): 2189.
Accessed on February 10, 2007, from the EbscoHOST database.

InChianti. "Association Between Vitamin D and Physical
Performance." *The Journal of Gerontology Series A: Biological
Sciences and Medical Sciences* 62(2007).

Jasnoski, M.L. and Kugler, J. "Relaxation, Imagery, and
Neuroimmunomodulation." Annals of the New York Academy
of Sciences. 496(1987):722-30. Accessed January 28, 2007 from
the EbscoHOST database.

Kash, P.M. and Lombard, J. *Freedom from Disease.* New York: St.
Martin's Press 2008.

Lee, J. and Hopkins, V. *What Your Doctor Will Not Tell You About
Menopause.* New York: Warner Books 2004.

Lutendorf, L., Logan, H., Kirchner, H.L., Rothrock, N., Svengalis,
S., and Iverson, K.L. "Effects of Relaxation and Stress on
the Capsaicin-Induced Local Inflammatory Response."

Psychosomatic Medicine 62(2000): 5. Accessed January 28, 2007 from the EbscoHOST database.

McKinney, C.H. "Effects of Guided Imagery and Music (GIM) Therapy on Mood and Corisol in Healthy Adults." *Health Psychology* 16(1997): 390-400.

Maguire, B.L. "The effects of Imagery on Attitudes and Moods in Multiple Sclerosis Patients." *Alternative Therapies in Health and Medicine* 2(1996): 75-9. Accessed February 10, 2007 from the EbscoHOST database.

Naparstek, B. *Invisible Heroes: Survivors of Trauma and How They Heal.* New York: Random House, Inc. 2004.

Pike, C., et al. "Testosterone Therapy May Prevent Alzheimer's Disease." *Science Daily* 20 Dec. 2006. http://www.sciencedaily. com/releases/2006/12/061219201939.htm

Resnick, S. and Scott Moffat. "Low Testosterone Levels Linked to Alzheimer's Disease in Older Men." *Journal of Neurology* (2007).

Schmidt, M. et al. "Prednisone Inhibits Clucocorticoid Dependent Aromatase Induction in Human Adipose Fibroblasts." *Journal of Endocrinology* 1589(1998): 401-7.

Schrauwan, P. and Westerstep, K. "The Role of High-Fat Diets and Physical Activity in the Regulation of Bodyweight." *The British Journal of Nutrition* 84(2000): 417-27.

Shambrook, C.J. "The Use of Single-Case Research Design to Investigate the Efficacy of Imagery Training." *Journal of Applied Sport Psychology* 8(1996): 2743. Retrieved February 10, 2007 from the EbscoHOST database.

Shin, B.S., et al. "Is Decreased Serum Testosterone Level a Risk Factor for Prostate Cancer? A Cohort Study of Korean Men." *Korean J Urology* 51(2010): 819-23. Accessed December, 2010 http://dx.doi.ort/10.4111/kju.2010.51.12.819.

Short, S.E., Smiley, M., and Ross-Stewart, L. "The Relationship Between Efficacy Beliefs and Imagery Use in Coaches." *Sport Psychologist* 19(2005): 380-394.

Smith, A.M., et al. "Testosterone Does Not Adversley Affect Fibrinogin or Tissue Plasminogen Activator (tPA) and Plasminogen Activator Inhibitor-1 (PAI-1) Levels in 46 Men with Chronic Angina." *European Journal of Endocrinology* 152(2005): 285-291.

Takai, N., Yamaguchi, M., Aragaki, T., Eto, K., Uchihashi, K. and Nishkawa, Y. "Effect of Psychological Stress on the Salivary Corisol and Amylase Levels in Healthy Young Adults." *Archives of Oral Biology* 49(2004): 963-8.

Watanabe, E., Fukuda, S., Hara, H., Maeda, Y., Ohira, H., and Shirakawa, T. "Differences in Relaxation by Means of Guided Imagery in a Healthy Community Sample." *Alternative Therapies* 12(2006): 60-66.

Whitaker, J. *Health and Healing.* 7(2007).

Wiegardt, P. A. "The Effect of Visual Imagery Perspective on the Learning, Retention, and Transfer of a Complex Field Hockey Skill. *"Dissertation Abstracts International Section A: Humanities and Social Sciences* 58(1998): 4697. Accessed February 10, 2007 from the EbscoHOST database.

Wilson, D. *Wilson's Thyroid (Temperature) Syndrome: A Reversible Low Temperature Problem.* Cornerstone Publishing, 1992.

Wilson, J.L. *Adrenal Fatigue: The 21st Century Stress Syndrome.* National Book Network: Lanham, 2008.

Huang, X. "Low LDL, Statin Use, and Parkinson's Disease, Another Benefit for Statins or Potential Harm." University of North Carolina Chapel Hill, 2007.

Zubrod, G., et al. "Novel Biochemical Markers of Cardiovascular Risk" *Emergency Medicine* (2006).

About the Author

Alan J. Sault, MD ABHM seeks to integrate the resources of traditional western medicine and holistic healing. He brings to his work forty years of experience in emergency and family medicine, and is a founding diplomate of the American Board of Holistic Medicine. He believes in the primacy of a doctor/patient partnership founded on trust and mutual respect. He brings together the wisdom of ancient healing with the practice of contemporary healing arts within the totality of mind, body and spirit, to create healing and prevent dis-ease.

He teaches workshops in stress management, andropause and menopause, Metabolic Syndrome, and anti-aging strategies in partnership with his wife, Jennifer Sault, MFA, MS/Eds, LMHC. In addition to his workshops, Alan is an accomplished archer and his writing on archery has been published *The Traditional Archer Magazine* of England. Alan and Jennifer make their home in Sarasota, Florida.